Core Topics in Thoracic Anesthesia

Core Topics in Thoracic Anesthesia

Edited by

CAIT P. SEARL

SAMEENA T. AHMED

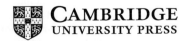
CAMBRIDGE
UNIVERSITY PRESS

CAMBRIDGE UNIVERSITY PRESS
Cambridge, New York, Melbourne, Madrid, Cape Town, Singapore, São Paulo, Delhi

Cambridge University Press
The Edinburgh Building, Cambridge CB2 8RU, UK

Published in the United States of America by Cambridge University Press, New York

www.cambridge.org
Information on this title: www.cambridge.org/9780521867122

First published 2009

Printed in the United Kingdom at the University Press, Cambridge

A catalog record for this publication is available from the British Library

Library of Congress Cataloguing in Publication data
Core topics in thoracic anesthesia / [edited by] Cait P. Searl, Sameena T. Ahmed.
    p. ; cm.
  Includes bibliographical references and index.
  ISBN 978-0-521-86712-2
  1. Anesthesia.   2. Chest – Surgery.   I. Searl, Cait P.   II. Ahm, Sameena T.
  [DNLM: 1. Anesthesia – methods.   2. Thoracic Surgical Procedures.   3. Thoracic
Diseases – surgery.   4. Thorax – drug effects.
  WF 980 C797   2009]

  RD536.C67   2009
  617.9′6 – dc22   2009005513

ISBN 978-0-521-86712-2 hardback

For Ben

Contents

SECTION 3 Post-operative management

Contributors

Sameena T. Ahmed
Freeman Hospital
Newcastle upon Tyne
UK

Douglas Aitchison
Essex Cardiothoracic Centre
Basildon and Thurrock University Hospital
Nethermayne
Basildon
UK

Abdalla Banni
Freeman Hospital
Newcastle upon Tyne
UK

Sion Barnard
Freeman Hospital
Newcastle upon Tyne
UK

Stephen Clark
Freeman Hospital
Newcastle upon Tyne
UK

Ian Conacher
Freeman Hospital
Newcastle upon Tyne
UK

Taj Dhallu
University Hospital of Wales
Cardiff
UK

Vijay Jeganath
University Hospital of North Staffordshire
Stoke-on-Trent
UK

John Jerstice
University Hospital of North Staffordshire
Stoke-on-Trent
UK

David Morrice
New Cross Hospital
Wolverhampton
UK

Tim Murphy
Freeman Hospital
Newcastle upon Tyne
UK

Jayanta Nandi
Surgical (Cardiothoracic) SPR
West Midlands Deanery
Department of Cardiothoracic Surgery
New Cross Hospital
Wolverhampton
UK

Alexander Ng
Heart & Lung Centre, New Cross Hospital
Wolverhampton
UK

Leena Pardeshi
Freeman Hospital
Newcastle upon Tyne
UK

David Place
University Hospital of Wales
Cardiff
UK

Mahesh Prabhu
Freeman Hospital
Newcastle upon Tyne
UK

O. P. Sanjay
Freeman Hospital
Newcastle upon Tyne
UK

Cait P. Searl
Freeman Hospital
Newcastle upon Tyne
UK

David C. Smith
Southampton General Hospital
Southampton
UK

Jonathan Hayden Smith
Freeman Hospital
Newcastle upon Tyne
UK

Christine Tan
University Hospital of Wales
Cardiff
UK

Kamen Valchanov
Papworth Hospital
Cambridge
UK

Alain Vuylsteke
Papworth Hospital
Cambridge
UK

Christopher Wigfield
Freeman Hospital
Newcastle upon Tyne
UK

Preface

This book is aimed primarily at trainees gaining experience in thoracic anesthesia. The content has been dictated both by what we would wish our trainees to gain from our own experience and practice and what we might expect them to know already! Acknowledgments and thanks are therefore due to the many patients who come under our care, who, together with our colleagues, have provided the basis for our experience and practice. We would also like to thank Cambridge University Press for their patience and support during the evolution of this text.

Abbreviations

ALI	acute lung injury	ISHLT	International Society of Heart and Lung Transplantation
ARDS	adult respiratory distress syndrome		
BPF	bronchopleural fistula	IRV	inspiratory reserve volume
BSLT	bilateral lung transplant	LVRS	lung volume reduction surgery
BTS	British Thoracic Society	LTx	lung transplant
CMV	cytomegalovirus	MPAP	mean pulmonary arterial pressure
CNS	central nervous system	MVV	minute ventilatory volume
CO	carbon monoxide	NIV	non-invasive ventilation
CO_2	carbon dioxide	NO	nitric oxide
COPD	chronic obstructive pulmonary disease	O_2	oxygen
cPAP	continuous positive airways pressure	OLV	one-lung ventilation
CPB	cardiopulmonary bypass	Pa	partial pressure (arterial)
CT	computerized tomography	P_A	partial pressure (alveolar)
CTEPH	chronic thromboembolic pulmonary hypertension	Pv	partial pressure (venous)
		PA	pulmonary artery
CVP	central venous pressure	PEA	pulmonary endarterectomy
CXR	chest X-ray	PEEP	positive end-expiratory pressure
DLT	double lumen endobronchial tube	PEF	peak expiratory flow
ECG	electrocardiogram	POD	post-operative delirium
ECMO	extracorporeal membrane oxygenation	Q	perfusion
ERV	expiratory reserve volume	RB	rigid bronchoscope
FEV_1	forced expiratory volume for 1 second	RV	residual volume
FOB	fiberoptic bronchoscope	TCB	torque control blocker
FRC	functional residual capacity	TLC	total lung capacity
FVC	forced vital capacity	TIVA	total intravenous anesthesia
GERD	gastro-esophageal reflux disease	TOE	transesophageal echocardiography
HPV	hypoxic pulmonary vasoconstriction	TV	tidal volume
I:E	inspired:expiratory time	V	ventilation
IPPV	intermittent positive pressure ventilation	VATS	video-assisted thoracoscopic surgery
		VC	vital capacity

Section 1 Pre-operative considerations

Chapter 1

Thoracic anatomy

DAVID MORRICE

The knowledge of certain aspects of thoracic anatomical arrangements is of great importance to the thoracic anesthetist. It assists in the correct positioning of endobronchial tubes, the identification of diseased lobes, in an understanding of the proposed surgery and also the potential complications that might occur. The availability of computerized tomography (CT) also means that the anesthetist can utilize this to his/her advantage in predicting difficulties in major cases. However, to interpret these, an understanding of normal anatomy is a prerequisite.

Tracheal, bronchial, lobar division

The course and division of the airway is readily seen on flexible and rigid bronchoscopy.

Trachea

This conduit for air and exhaled gases arises from the lower border of the larynx at approximately the level of cervical vertebra C6. The trachea descends in line with the vertebra and moves slightly to the right and posteriorly in doing so. It consists of 16–20 C-shaped cartilaginous rings that provide a semi-rigid structure. Posteriorly the longitudinal trachealis muscle (non-striated) completes the tube structure. This muscle layer has the appearance of a flowing river and provides an easy landmark to orientation when performing a fiberoptic bronchoscopy. Bifurcation occurs at the level of thoracic vertebra T4. Thus the average length of the trachea in an adult male is 15 cm. The usual anterioposterior diameter is 20 mm.

Throughout its course the esophagus lies directly behind the trachea, with the recurrent laryngeal nerves lying in the groove in between. In the upper (extra thoracic) trachea, the isthmus of the thyroid overlies the trachea anteriorly with the thyroid lobes lying laterally. The relations of the trachea are shown in Figure 1.1. Moving down into the thoracic cavity the thymus overlies the trachea not far below the sternal notch, and below this are arterial vessels arising from the aorta below. These are from right to left, the brachiocephalic artery, left carotid, and below this the ascending aorta arches in front of the trachea, giving in addition to the above the left common carotid and subclavian arteries. During mediastinoscopy the brachiocephalic artery may be compressed by the rigid bronchoscope, affecting the blood supply to the right arm. The medial aspect of the right upper lobe lies against the trachea. The recurrent laryngeal nerves innervate the upper trachea.

Core Topics in Thoracic Anesthesia, ed. Cait P. Searl and Sameena T. Ahmed. Published by Cambridge University Press.

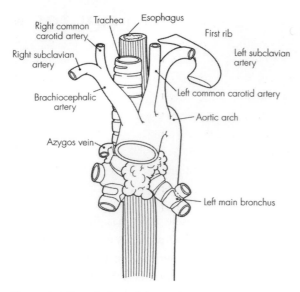

Figure 1.1 The relations of the trachea.

The bronchi and bronchial tree

The bronchial tree with its divisions is illustrated in Figure 1.2.

The carina and surrounding structures

The last tracheal ring is larger and wider than the others, forming a sharp sagittal ridge called the carina (Latin for the keel of a boat). The carina marks the bifurcation into right and left bronchi. Several important tracheobronchial lymph nodes lie within close proximity and tumor spread to these nodes may blunt the sharp edge of the carina. In addition mediastinoscopy to biopsy these nodes will reveal the intimate relations of the pulmonary artery, aorta and branches and superior vena cava. The pulmonary artery is particularly at risk of injury during this procedure.

Right and left bronchi

The right main bronchus compared to the left is shorter and descends more vertically, i.e. at 25° compared to 45°. This leads to a tendency for endo-bronchial tubes to favor entry to the right. It ends

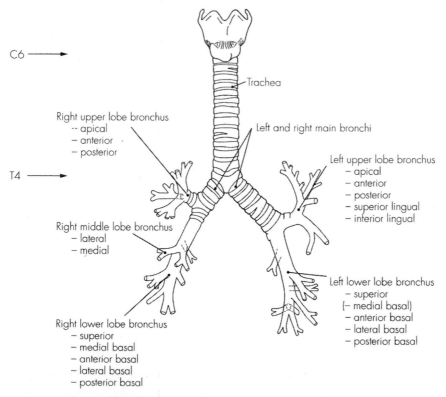

Figure 1.2 The bronchial tree.

when the right upper lobe orifice branches out after 2.5 cm. This lobe consists of three segments (apical, anterior and posterior).

The right upper lobe orifice is directed at 90° from the right main bronchus and may need some bronchoscopic maneuvering to visualize. The apical segment is directed vertically (the other two horizontally); hence on a "slice" of CT it appears as a small well-defined circle. This can be used to aid the localization of tumors within the lungs. Occasionally this lobe may arise higher, even from the trachea.

Following this first division the main bronchus continues as the bronchus intermedius for 3 cm until the middle lobe branches in a direction medially and downwards. Two segments are contained in the medial lobe (lateral and medial) which both project horizontally. This medial lobe is anteriorly placed and wedged between the anterior segment of the upper lobe and the anterior basal segment of the lower lobe.

Thereafter the main bronchus supplies the lower lobe. First to branch off horizontally, opposite the medial lobe orifice, is the apical segment of the lower lobe, worth mentioning because it is directed posteriorly. It is thus prone to collecting secretions in the supine patient. Four further branches are made in a downward direction, all to basal segments of the lower lobe. Thus the right medial lobe and apical portion of the right lower lobe divide at a similar level and appear as a row of three orifices, sometimes being referred to as the secondary carina.

On the **left side** the bronchial divisions supply the left upper lobe, lingula and lower lobe. At about 5 cm from the carina, the upper lobe bronchus branches to supply both the upper lobe and the lingula. The upper lobe bronchus is 1 cm long and supplies apical, anterior and posterior segments. The upper lobe is difficult to inspect due to its vertical take off and the anterior and posterior segments are also vertically orientated. The lingular orifice appears more in line with the left main bronchus (i.e. obliquely), and its bronchus is 2–3 cm long. It divides into two segments, superior and inferior, which also head in an oblique direction. In a similar fashion to the right middle lobe, the lingula is anteriorly placed and wedged between anterior segments of the left upper and lower lobes. The left lower lobe bronchus is directed downwards with division firstly into an apical segment arising from the posterior wall and directed horizontally. Below this the bronchus heads vertically downwards and divides into anterior, lateral and posterior basal branches.

Importance of bronchopulmonary segments

There are 20 segments as described above and each can be considered as being discrete physiologically functional units, as each segment has its own separate arterial supply, and venous and lymphatic drainage. The divisions are further illustrated in Figure 1.3. In the case of a lobectomy e.g. for neoplasia the surgeon will have to ensure correct isolation of each of these vessel types to avoid venous congestion or ischemia of other parts of the lung. As a rule each segment is pyramidal shaped and will receive a single branch of the pulmonary artery to perfuse the alveoli. These follow the course of the bronchi, and the division into bronchioles. The bronchus for each segment divides about 15 times into terminal bronchioles. Blood from each segment is drained by intersegmental veins that lie in the connective tissue around the segment, which generally leads to a single branch from each segment. However, the right upper lobe often has additional draining branches of the pulmonary vein. Lymphatics tend to closely follow the course of the bronchi. These drain into tracheobronchial lymph nodes located at the bifurcation of the larger bronchi.

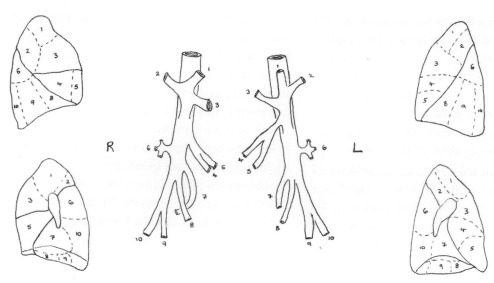

Figure 1.3 The bronchopulmonary segments.

Alveolar units

The terminal bronchioles further divide into respiratory bronchioles from which alveoli arise, finally ending in sacs of alveoli. Deoxygenated blood from the tissues is pumped forward from the right heart via the pulmonary arteries and intrasegmental branches to the fine capilliary beds around the alveolar sacs. Here, as described elsewhere, O_2 and CO_2 gas exchange occurs. Thereafter oxygenated blood drains into the pulmonary vein system, which collects in the intersegmental septa and drains ultimately into the left atrium.

Bronchial arteries

These smaller vessels supply the stroma of the lung including the bronchi, pleura and nodes. They follow the posterior aspect of the bronchi as they divide. There are usually two left bronchial arteries arising from the descending thoracic aorta and a right arising variably from the aorta or intercostal arteries. Bronchial veins drain only the more proximal bronchial divisions and may be susceptible to compression by edema as they cross the bronchial wall.

The hilum

The structures that enter the lung are the pulmonary arteries, veins, the primary bronchi, pulmonary nerve plexi and bronchial arteries. Where these structures enter and leave the lung is termed the hilum.

The pleura

Each pleural sac is a closed cavity lined by a serous membrane invaginated by a lung. The outer wall of the chest is lined by the parietal pleura while the visceral pleura cover the lung. The layers of pleura are continuous around the root of the lung. The parietal pleura lines the ribs, costal cartilages and the intercostal spaces, extending superiorly beyond the thoracic inlet to form the cervical dome of pleura. Inferiorly it forms a narrow gutter around the margin of the diaphragm, the costodiaphragmatic recess, and similarly anteriorly in front of the heart, the left costal and mediastinal surfaces are in contact forming the costomediastinal recess. The pleura is supplied by blood from the tissues it covers. The visceral pleura has no pain fibers but the parietal pleura has a rich nerve supply from nerves in adjacent tissues. The lymphatic drainage of the visceral pleura is to a superficial plexus in the lung and then to hilar nodes, and the parietal pleura drains to parasternal, diaphragmatic and posterior mediastinal nodes.

The paravertebral space

The borders of the thoracic paravertebral space are imprecise. It is a wedge-shaped space with its base being formed by the lateral surface of the vertebral body and intervertebral foramen. It is thought that the prevertebral fascia and anterior longitudinal ligament usually form a barrier to communication to the contralateral paravertebral space, breached only by lymphatic channels. The posterior wall is formed by the inner surface of the vertebral transverse process, the neck of the rib and the attached superior costotransverse ligament. The lateral boundary is formed by the ribs and internal intercostal muscles. The anterior wall is the parietal pleura.

The diaphragm

The diaphragm is a musculotendinous septum separating the thoracic and abdominal cavities. It consists of a peripheral muscular part attached to the edges of a central trilobed tendon (see Figure 1.4).

The peripheral muscular part is divisible into three sections by its attachments:

1. Sternal part – from the back of the xiphoid process by two muscular slips.
2. Costal part – from the inner surfaces of the lower six ribs and costal cartilages, interdigitating with transverse abdominis.
3. Vertebral part – from the sides of the bodies of the upper lumbar vertebrae by two crura and from the medial and lateral arcuate ligaments on each side. The right crus is attached to the bodies of the first three vertebrae and the left crus to the first two. The larger right crus passes forwards and to the right surrounding the esophageal opening. The medial arcuate ligament is the thickened upper edge of the psoas fascia and passes from the body of the first lumbar vertebra to its transverse process. The lateral arcuate ligament is anterior to quadratus lumborum passing from the transverse process of the 1st lumbar vertebra to the 12th rib.

The two halves of the diaphragm are supplied by the corresponding phrenic nerves. The periphery also receives additional sensory branches from

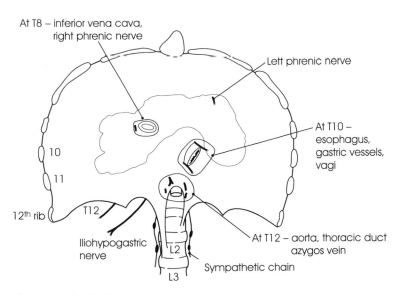

Figure 1.4 The diaphragm.

intercostal nerves. There are three large openings in the diaphragm from before forwards: for the inferior vena cava (with the right phrenic nerve) in the central tendon to the right of the midline at the level of the 8th thoracic vertebra; for the esophagus at the level of T10 as above (with branches of the vagus nerve and esophageal branches of the left gastric vessels); and for the aorta, between the crura of the diaphragm in front of T12. This also transmits the thoracic duct and azygous vein. The left phrenic nerve pierces the left dome of the diaphragm.

FURTHER READING

- Erdmann A. *Concise Anatomy for Anaesthetists*. Cambridge: Cambridge University Press, 2002.
- Cornley DM, Rosse C. *Interactive Atlas of Thoracic Viscera*. University of Washington, 1996, accessed at www9.biostr.washington-edu.

Chapter 2

Respiratory physiology

CAIT P. SEARL

The primary task of the lungs is respiration. Respiration is the exchange of gases between an organism and its environment with the utilization of O_2 and production of CO_2. In a multicellular organism such as man, diffusion pathways are too long for the rapid delivery of O_2 and removal of CO_2. The circulating blood provides a transport system to carry the respiratory gases between the lungs and the distant cells. Oxygen in the inspired air reaches the pulmonary alveoli (ventilation) where it diffuses into the blood whereas CO_2 diffuses in the opposite direction.

Respiratory mechanics

Bulk flow of air in and out of the lungs is achieved by pressure gradients between the mouth and alveoli. These pressure gradients are achieved by movement outward and inwards of the chest creating changes in pleural pressure and hence alveolar pressure changes. When the gas is stationary alveolar and mouth pressures are the same and at atmospheric pressure. Whether the air is flowing or not, the pleural pressure is affected by the inward elastic recoil of the lungs.

Inspiration is an active process: muscular contraction increases the volume of the chest, the lungs expand and the intrapulmonary pressure in the alveoli falls so that the air flows into the lungs. During expiration the lungs and chest recoil to the positions they occupied at the beginning of inspiration. Expiration is largely passive. During quiet breathing, the diaphragm accounts for around 75% of the lung volume change by its contraction during inspiration and relaxation during expiration. The diaphragm by itself or the scalene and external intercostal muscles alone can maintain adequate ventilation at rest. Expiration is achieved by passive recoil but can be assisted by contraction of the abdominal muscles and the internal intercostal muscles.

Respiratory volumes

The volume in the lungs at maximal inspiration is the total lung capacity (TLC; approximately 6 liters). Its subcomponents are inspiratory reserve volume (IRV), tidal volume, expiratory reserve volume (ERV) and residual volume (RV). The first three comprise the vital capacity (VC) and the latter two comprise the functional residual capacity (FRC) (see Table 2.1 and Figure 2.1). These volumes and capacities increase with body size and are smaller in females. There is a reduction in elastic recoil of the lungs and stiffening of the chest wall with aging. This leads to a gradual increase in RV and FRC and a fall in VC with little change in TLC.

Core Topics in Thoracic Anesthesia, ed. Cait P. Searl and Sameena T. Ahmed. Published by Cambridge University Press.
© Cambridge University Press 2009.

Table 2.1 Lung volumes and capacities.

Ventilatory volumes

Tidal volume (TV)	Amplitude of the oscillation in lung volume during quiet respiration, usually about 400–500 ml
Inspiratory reserve volume (IRV)	Maximum volume of air which can be inspired in excess of normal inspiration
Expiratory reserve volume (ERV)	Maximum volume of air which can be expired in excess of normal expiration
Residual volume (RV)	The volume of air remaining in the lungs after maximal expiration; $RV = FRC - ERV$

Lung capacities

Total lung capacity	Represents the sum of all the ventilatory volumes plus the residual volume
Vital capacity (VC)	The sum of the ventilatory volumes; the volume of gas that is expelled from the lungs from peak inspiration to peak expiration
Functional residual capacity (FRC)	Volume of gas left in the lungs at the end of quiet expiration
Inspiratory capacity	Equals tidal volume plus inspiratory reserve volume

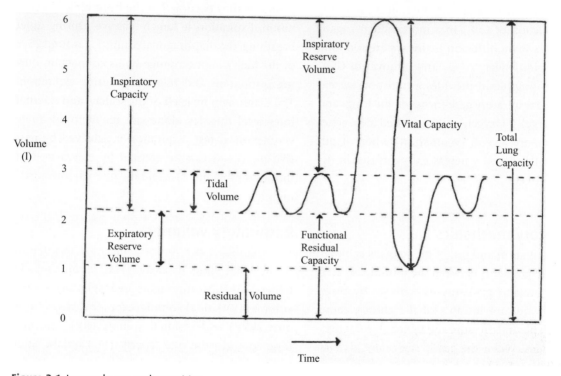

Figure 2.1 Lung volumes and capacities.

Lung compliance

Compliance is a measure of the difficulty of inflation of the lungs. It can be determined from the gradient of a plot of lung volume against distending pressure. This relationship demonstrates hysteresis but an average compliance can be determined using a linear interpolation (see Figure 2.2).

The most important physiological measure is the compliance of the intact respiratory system (i.e. the compliance of the lung and chest wall together). This is usually about $11\,\text{kPa}^{-1}$ ($100\,\text{ml/cm}\;H_2O$). This may be reduced by diseases of the lung such as pulmonary fibrosis or by abnormalities of the chest wall.

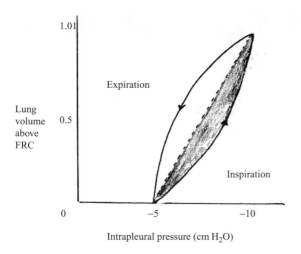

Figure 2.2 Compliance of the lungs.

Dead space

Gas exchange in the respiratory system only occurs in the alveoli. The part of the airway that does not participate in gas exchange is called the dead space. The total dead space consists of the "anatomical" dead space and the "physiological" dead space. The "anatomical" dead space consists of the mouth, nose, pharynx, trachea and main bronchi, and is equivalent to approximately 150 ml. The anatomical dead space functions as a conduit in which the air is filtered of dust particles, humidified and warmed. The functional dead space is normally equivalent to the anatomical dead space. If alveoli are ventilated but no gas exchange is taking place,

then these contribute to the functional dead space. The volume of total dead space can be calculated from the CO_2 content of alveolar gas and the tidal volume using the Bohr equation (Box 2.1).

Gas exchange in the lungs

The movement of O_2 and CO_2 in and out of the capillaries both in the lungs and in the peripheral tissues depends on gas diffusion. This in turn is affected by three main factors:
1. The partial pressure gradients of each gas.
2. The diffusion coefficient for each gas.
3. The physical properties of the tissues at the site of exchange (surface area, diffusion distances).

The lungs are well adapted for gas diffusion with a large alveolar surface area and a very thin layer of fluid and tissue separating alveolar gas from pulmonary blood.

Ventilation:perfusion ratio

Normal gas exchange requires both that the alveoli are adequately ventilated and that they are adequately perfused. This relationship is quantified by the alveolar:perfusion ratio, V/Q. V/Q = alveolar ventilation rate/pulmonary blood flow. When this deviates from normal, ventilation-perfusion mismatch occurs. If an area of the lung is inadequately ventilated but adequately perfused, V/Q will be reduced. Blood passing through such areas will be inadequately oxygenated reducing the partial pressure of O_2 in the systemic arterial blood: physiological shunting of blood. This is a major factor contributing to the abnormal blood gases seen in many respiratory diseases.

Pulmonary blood flow

Virtually all the cardiac output passes through the lungs, at arterial pressures of about one-sixth of systemic. The overall pulmonary blood volume is about 500 ml but only 80 ml is in the capillaries. Pulmonary vascular pressures are mainly influenced by gravity. When in the erect position,

---

Box 2.1 The Bohr equation

$$V_D = \frac{V_T(F_{A_{CO_2}} - F_{E_{CO_2}})}{F_{A_{CO_2}}}$$

Where
  V_D is the functional dead space
  V_T is the tidal volume
  $F_A CO_2$ is the fractional CO_2 concentration in the alveolar gas (can be determined from the terminal portion of air expired)
  $F_E CO_2$ is the fractional CO_2 concentration in the expired gas

11

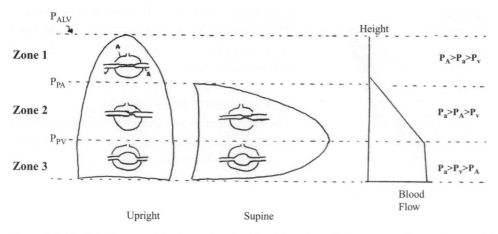

Figure 2.3 The 'West' zones of the lungs showing blood flow through the erect and supine lung and the influence of gravity.

blood flow is nearly zero at the apex and greatest at the bases (see Figure 2.3) as defined by West. This variation is greater than the similar variation in ventilation, resulting in the highest ventilation:perfusion ratio at the top of the lungs. This remains largely true whether the body is supine, prone or in lateral position rather than upright – the zones remaining from uppermost down as depicted. When lying down or in lateral decubitus position zone 1 may not apply as the height is not sufficient.

Hypoxic pulmonary vasoconstriction

Hypoxic pulmonary vasoconstriction continues to attract interest because of persistent mystery about its biochemical mechanism (Box 2.2) and its exact physiological function. Recent work suggests an important role for pulmonary arteriolar smooth muscle cell oxygen-sensitive voltage-dependent potassium channels. Inhibition of these channels by decreased PO_2 inhibits outward potassium current, causing membrane depolarization, and calcium entry through voltage-dependent calcium channels. Endothelium-derived vasoconstricting and vasodilating mediators modulate this intrinsic smooth muscle cell reactivity to hypoxia. Hypoxic pulmonary vasoconstriction seems to decrease with

age, and exhibits marked inter-species and inter-individual differences. The magnitude of HPV in vivo is inversely proportional to lung segment size. The main determinant of HPV is the alveolar partial pressure of O_2, but mixed venous O_2 contributes to approximately one fifth of the response.

Box 2.2 Hypoxic pulmonary vasoconstriction

HPV is inhibited by
- mediators e.g. Substance P; Calcitonin; atrial natriuretic peptide
- endothelium-derived vasodilators e.g. prostacyclin; nitric oxide
- α-adrenergic blockade
- β-adrenergic stimulation
- increased left atrial pressure
- increased alveolar pressure
- alkalosis
- peripheral chemoreceptor stimulation
- vasodilating drugs e.g. calcium channel blockers; halogenated anesthetics.

HPV is enhanced by
- acidosis
- β-adrenergic blockade
- epidural blockade
- low dose serotonin
- inhibition of cyclo-oxygenase (aspirin, NSAIDs)
- inhibition of NO synthase (L-arginine analogs).

Control of respiration

Respiration is controlled in the central nervous system with voluntary breathing managed by the cortex and autonomic respiration by structures in the medullopontine region. Efferent output from these two sources is integrated by the spinal cord. Control of automatic breathing is governed by centers in the pons and medulla. These modulate the depth and rate of inspiration. Appropriate blood levels of O_2, CO_2 and hydrogen ions (pH) are maintained through adjustments of respiration through the medullary center as it responds to afferent inputs from receptors. The medullary center is also important in the maintenance of respiratory rhythm and for the Hering–Breuer reflex, which inhibits respiration when the lungs are stretched. Other inputs to the medullary center include:

- Proprioceptors – coordinating respiration with muscular activity.
- Body temperature.
- Higher CNS centers (cortex, limbic system, hypothalamus) influencing breathing, during, for example, pain, anxiety and sneezing.
- Presso- or baroceptors – also feeding into the cardioinhibitory area.

Voluntary breath holding inhibits automatic respiration until the break point is reached when the rise in $PaCO_2$ and fall in PaO_2 override the voluntary inhibition. This breakpoint can be delayed by prior hyperventilation.

In patients with chronic CO_2 retention, the medullary center becomes insensitive to changes in $PaCO_2$ so that the PaO_2 is the chief driver of respiration. This is the group of patients in whom breathing 100% O_2 could abolish respiratory drive, eventually causing coma and death. This is relatively uncommon and should not be used as a reason not to administer oxygen.

Non-respiratory functions

Some of the non-respiratory functions are listed below.

- The pulmonary capillary bed acts as a blood filter by removing small clots, detached cells and air bubbles before they reach the systemic system.
- The pulmonary blood vessels act as a reservoir for blood.
- The airways remove airborne particles by a combination of phagocytosis and mucociliary action together with coughing.
- Ventilation of the airways contributes to heat loss and water loss.
- Lung tissue has many metabolic functions, including:
  Conversion of angiotensin I to angiotensin II;
  Synthesis and removal of bradykinin and prostaglandins;
  Storage and release of serotonin and histamine;
  Inactivation of norepinephrine and epinephrine;
  Secretion of heparin by mast cells and immunoglobulins in bronchial mucosa;
  Synthesis of peptides including substance P and opiates.

Effects of anesthesia on respiratory physiology

Under general anesthesia and in the supine position, forced vital capacity (FVC) is reduced by around a fifth in an adult. Obesity and multiple other causes may also further reduce the FVC. A large enough decrease in FVC may bring the end-expiratory volumes below the closing volumes. Closing volumes are the volumes at which small airways begin to close. When the small airways begin to close, areas of low V/Q mismatch develop.

Physiology of spontaneous ventilation in the lateral decubitus position

General anesthesia will reduce the compliance of both upper and lower lungs. This can be returned towards normal by the application of positive end-expiratory pressure (PEEP). The weight of the mediastinum and the pressure of the abdominal contents on the diaphragm can impair lower lung expansion and causes decreased FVC. However the greater curvature of the diaphragm will also result in more efficient contraction, with greater expansion matching increased blood flow to the dependent lung. The result is that V/Q remains matched.

During spontaneous ventilation the dependent diaphragm will move towards the head end during expiration, pushing the mediastinum upwards. This produces inefficient ventilation. The resulting mediastinal shift also reduces perfusion because of reduced venous return secondary to sympathetic activation. If the upper chest wall is opened during spontaneous ventilation, paradoxical respiration occurs. During inspiration, gases are drawn out of the upper lung causing it to collapse. During expiration, gases pass from the bottom lung to the upper lung causing it to inflate. This paradoxical respiration causes mediastinal shift generating more work.

Physiology of two-lung ventilation in the lateral decubitus position

Positive pressure ventilation results in most of the ventilation being directed into the upper rather than the lower lung. As perfusion remains greatest in the lower lung, ventilation–perfusion mismatch increases. The result in an anesthetized patient with a closed chest in the lateral decubitus position is a non-dependent lung that is poorly perfused but well ventilated, and a dependent lung that is well perfused but poorly ventilated. Opening the chest wall and pleural space does not change the perfusion distribution but may have a significant effect in terms of ventilation. In the paralyzed, ventilated

anesthetized patient, the non-dependent lung is no longer confined making it easier to ventilate and consequently over-ventilated and under-perfused worsening the mismatch.

Physiology of one-lung ventilation in lateral decubitus position

The blood flow gradient due to gravity favors the dependent lung during one-lung ventilation (OLV). If the non-dependent lung is not ventilated any blood flow to it becomes shunt flow. This will result in a larger alveolar-to-arterial oxygen tension difference with a lower PaO_2 for a given oxygen concentration under identical circumstances, when compared to two-lung ventilation in the same position. In contrast OLV has much less of an effect on $PaCO_2$ than on the PaO_2. The blood flowing through the relatively under-ventilated alveoli will retain more CO_2 and not take up O_2. As the CO_2 dissociation curve is relatively linear in the physiological range, this favors elimination of CO_2 and the maintenance of relatively normocapnia despite OLV. The O_2 dissociation curve is relatively flat at the top end of the sigmoid-shaped curve and so less of an increase is possible in the uptake of O_2. Hence while the ventilated lung is able to eliminate sufficient CO_2 to compensate for the non-ventilated lung, it is unable to take up sufficient O_2 to compensate in the same way.

FURTHER READING

- West JB. *Respiratory Physiology: The Essentials*, 7th edn. Philadelphia, PA: Lippincott Williams & Wilkins, 2004.
- Guyton WF. *Review of Medical Physiology*, 22nd edn. New York: Lange Medical/McGraw-Hill, 2005.

Chapter 3

Respiratory pharmacology

CAIT P. SEARL

The twin requirements of respiration (ventilation and perfusion) result in the lungs both being exposed to the external environment and the internal environment through the bloodstream. This is utilized in the uptake, accumulation and metabolism of both environmental and blood-borne "foreign" substances including drugs and environmental pollutants. The importance of the lungs in the pharmokinetics of many drugs is often forgotten. There are several metabolic pathways known to be present in the endothelial tissues: the cytochrome P-450 monooxygenase enzymes are likely to be particularly important. Many of the drugs that we use as anesthetists are metabolized in the lungs including sympathomimetics, antihistamines, opiates and local anesthetics (Box 3.1).

A thoracic anesthetist needs to be familiar with the drugs that "respiratory" patients are likely to be receiving and also with their potential use in aid of anesthesia and post-operative management. It is also useful to be aware of potential effects of the drugs that we utilize in anesthesia on the respiratory system.

Drugs active in the respiratory tract
Drugs used in the treatment of asthma and bronchospasm

Asthma is clinically characterized by recurrent episodes of coughing, wheezing and dyspnea. It is characterized by increased responsiveness of the trachea and bronchi to various stimuli and by widespread airway narrowing. The pathology consists of contraction of airway smooth muscle and mucosal thickening from edema and cellular infiltration. Bronchospasm results from a combination of a release of mediators and an exaggerated response to their effects. Therapy is directed at relaxing the airway smooth muscle, reducing bronchial responsiveness and preventing mast cell degranulation.

BRONCHODILATORS
1. **Direct relaxants of respiratory smooth muscle** – methylxanthines such as theophylline; act by reducing the breakdown of cAMP through the inhibition of phosphodiesterases. Methylxanthines are administered orally or intravenously and can have a number of side-effects due to the increased concentration of cAMP in other systems, causing nervousness, tremor, diuretic activity; secretion of gastric acid; and positive chronotropic and inotropic effects. These compounds have a relatively narrow therapeutic range. They are no longer used as first-line therapy.
2. **Selective Beta$_2$ adrenergic agonists** – e.g. salbutamol, terbutaline. The β_2 agonists act

Core Topics in Thoracic Anesthesia, ed. Cait P. Searl and Sameena T. Ahmed. Published by Cambridge University Press.
© Cambridge University Press 2009.

Box 3.1 Compounds cleared/metabolized by the lungs

Adenosine
Amphetamine
Angiotensin I (converted to angiotensin II)
Atrial natriuretic peptides
Bradykinin
Bupivacaine
Chlorpromazine
Fentanyl
5-Hydroxytryptamine (serotonin)
Imipramine
Isoprenaline
Lidocaine
Metaramine
Methadone
Morphine
Norephidrine
Prostaglandin E_1, E_2 and F_{2a}
Steroids

Compounds released from the lung
Adenosine
Heparin
Histamine
5-Hydroxytryptamine
Leukotriene A_4, B_4, C_4, D_4 and E_4
NO
Plasminogen activator
Prostaglandin I_2, E and F

primarily on airway smooth muscle and are the most effective form of bronchodilator treatment.

3. **Anticholinergic agents** – muscarinic antagonists inhibit the effects of vagal-released acetylcholine at muscarinic receptors in the airways. Atropine is the classic muscarinic antagonist but systemically has no selectivity, limiting its usefulness. Ipratropium delivered by inhaler is poorly absorbed and so has few systemic side-effects. Although the onset can be delayed (up to 45 minutes), the effects are prolonged.

4. **Mast cell stabilizers** – The chromones (sodium chromoglycate and sodium nedocromil) act predominantly by stabilizing mast cells.

LEUKOTRIENE ANTAGONISTS

The cysteinyl leukotrienes cause smooth muscle constriction and proliferation and are important mediators in the inflammatory process. Montelukast and zafirlukast block the effects of cysteinyl leukotrienes in the airways through antagonizing their actions at leukotriene receptors. They are effective when used in asthma both alone and in addition to an inhaled corticosteroid, having an additive effect with the latter.

MAGNESIUM SULPHATE

Intravenous magnesium has been used to supplement the bronchodilatory effects of inhaled B_2 agonists.

GLUCOCORTICOID THERAPY

Inhaled corticosteroids are amongst the most important treatment agents for bronchospasm as they both increase the number of $beta_2$-adrenergic receptors and their responsiveness to stimulation. They also reduce mucous production and hypersecretion and inhibit the inflammatory response. Systemic glucocorticoid therapy may also be necessary both with acute severe attacks of bronchospasm and episodes of bronchospasm that are failing to respond to inhaled bronchodilators.

Relief of cough

Treatment of cough mainly consists of treatment of the underlying cause. A productive cough in general should not be suppressed as this may result in sputum retention. Cough remedies are categorized into antitussives and expectorants. Antitussive agents may be either centrally or peripherally acting. The centrally acting agents, including dextromethorphan and codeine, work by depressing the medullary cough center or associated higher centers. Peripherally acting agents may act on either the afferent or efferent side of the reflex pathway and include demulcents, local anesthetics, humidifying aerosols and steam inhalations. Inhalation of water containing volatile substances such as eucalyptus oil may via the deliberate inspiration of warm moist air provide symptomatic relief in bronchitis.

Mucolytics

Mucolytics are prescribed in order to facilitate expectoration by decreasing the viscosity of sputum. They have been shown to benefit some patients with chronic obstructive airways disease and chronic cough with a reduction in exacerbations of the condition. The treatment can be with oral therapy such as carbocisteine and methyl cysteine hydrochloride or by a nebulized route for example dornase alfa. This latter is mainly recommended for use in patients with cystic fibrosis.

Effects of drugs used during anesthesia on the respiratory system
Volatile anesthetics

Volatile anesthetic agents are mainly used for the maintenance of anesthesia during thoracic procedures. They cause a decrease in FRC through decreasing chest wall recoil, bronchodilation, inhibition of HPV and blunting of the ventilatory response to hypoxia. These effects mean post-operatively that any residual volatile anesthesia can cause significant impairment of lung function.

Opiates

Opiate drugs are usually necessary for the treatment of pain in association with thoracic surgery. All these drugs will cause respiratory depression although the magnitude of this effect is variable according to the individual drug and according to the timing of administration, route of administration and patient factors such as comorbidities.

Propofol

Propofol is often used to both induce and maintain anesthesia during thoracic procedures. It has a rapid onset and offset allowing rapid recovery. It has relatively little effect on HPV and no differences in intra-operative PaO_2 were demonstrated when compared with a volatile maintained anesthesia. Other comparisons with volatile anesthesia have shown that propofol is associated with less post-operative lung function impairment.

Other induction agents

Thiopentone remains a popular drug for induction of anesthesia. It is known to release histamine and has been associated with bronchospasm in asthmatic patients. In contrast **etomidate** rarely causes histamine release and is advocated by some as the drug to use in patients who are at risk of bronchospasm. It is however associated with adrenal suppression, specifically cortisol production from 11-deoxycortisol. **Ketamine** is not commonly used as an agent for induction in adults, but has bronchodilatory properties and has been used in the treatment of asthma. Benzodiazepines such as midazolam and diazepam will cause decreases in tidal volume although they are associated with an increase in respiratory rate. Both agents will decrease hypoxic ventilatory drive with only partial reversal by the antagonist flumazenil.

Muscle relaxants

Most neuromuscular relaxants have no direct drug effect on the lungs beyond the effects induced by muscle relaxation and paralysis. Some, notably atracurium and mivacurium, cause histamine release predominantly with hemodynamic consequences but also with effects on bronchomotor tone. Rocuronium, vecuronium and cisatracurium have relatively little cardiovascular or respiratory side-effects. The main concerns with usage of a muscle relaxant are ensuring that it is adequately reversed with no residual effect. Patients with respiratory disease are likely to be particularly sensitive to small decreases in respiratory muscle function secondary to residual muscle weakness. Reversal of neuromuscular blockade is usually assisted with the administration of neostigmine in combination with an anticholinergic agent such as atropine or glycopyrrolate. Even with the addition of the anticholinergic agent there may be a significant increase in airway resistance secondary to the inhibition of endogenous acetylcholine by neostigmine.

FURTHER READING

- Boer F. Drug handling by the lungs. *Br J Anaesth* 2003; **91**: 50.
- Mora CT, Torjman M, White P. Effects of diazepam and flumazenil on sedation and hypoxic ventilator drive. *Anesth Analg* 1989; **68**: 473−478.
- Speicher A, Jessberger J, Braun R, *et al.* Postoperative pulmonary function following lung surgery. *Anaesthetist* 1995; **44**: 265.
- Spies C, Zuane V, Pauli MH, *et al.* A comparison of Enflurane and propofol in thoracic surgery. *Anaesthetist* 1991; **40**: 14.

Chapter 4

Respiratory diseases

CAIT P. SEARL

In this chapter, common respiratory disease processes will be reviewed. The aim is to give an overview of the disorders that may be met by the thoracic anesthetist and where relevant to consider their anesthetic implications.

Infective disorders
Pneumonia

Pneumonia is defined as infection of the lower respiratory tract parenchyma by infectious agents such as bacteria, viruses and fungi. Pneumonitis is an inflammation of the lung parenchyma caused by non-infectious causes including chemicals, radiation and autoimmune diseases.

The commonest mechanism triggering pneumonia is upper airway colonization with potentially pathogenic organisms that are subsequently aspirated. However the oropharynx may be colonized with such organisms in normal health and the presence of such organisms is not always sufficient to implicate them in the disease process. Pneumonia is the result of a complex interaction between the patient, the infecting organism and the environment. Important factors are the virulence of the causative organism and the vulnerability of the patient. Age and the previous state of health of the patient influence the probability of different causative agents. The likely causes of pneumo-

nia in differing clinical circumstances are shown in Box 4.1.

Patients with pneumonia may present with a history of cough, production of purulent sputum and fever, together with pleuritic chest pain and shortness of breath. The presence of localized chest signs on examination such as crackles or bronchial breathing suggests pneumonia but may not always be present. The severity of pneumonia can be assessed using a scoring system such as the CURB-65 severity score as shown in Box 4.2. The investigations necessary will depend on the severity of the pneumonia: patients with a mild illness responding rapidly to antibiotics do not usually require further investigation whereas more extensive investigations are indicated for patients requiring admission to hospital. A chest X-ray will confirm diagnosis by demonstrating consolidation (Figure 4.1). It may also be helpful in detecting complications such as lung abscess or empyema (see Chapter 17). More specific investigations are aimed at identifying the causative agent – for example, sputum culture $+/-$ a Gram stain; antigen detection tests and serological tests. *Streptococcus pneumonia* is the most common cause of community-acquired pneumonia, but atypical pathogens such as *Mycoplasma pneumonia* are also frequent, so treatment is often with a combination of amoxicillin and a macrolide

Core Topics in Thoracic Anesthesia, ed. Cait P. Searl and Sameena T. Ahmed. Published by Cambridge University Press.
© Cambridge University Press 2009.

Box 4.1 Likely causes of pneumonia

- Previously well infant
  Respiratory synctial virus
  Adenovirus
  Bacterial
- Previously ill infant
  Staphylococcus
  E. coli
  Viral agents
- Children
  Viruses
  Pneumococcus
  Mycoplasma
- Adults
  Pneumococcus
  Mycoplasma
  H. influenzae
  Viruses
  Staphylococcus
  Legionella
- Adults with concurrent respiratory illnesses; the elderly and debilitated
  Pneumococcus
  H. influenzae
  Staphylococcus
  Klebsiella
  Consider tuberculosis; *Legionella*; underlying tumor
- Immunocompromised adults
  Pneumocystis pneumonia
  Cytomegalovirus
  Adenovirus
  Herpes simplex
  Bacteria (*Legionella, Staphylococcus, Pneumococcus*)
  Opportunistic mycobacteria; tuberculosis
- Hospital-acquired pneumonia in adults
  Gram-negative bacteria (*Pseudomonas, Klebsiella, Proteus*)
  Staphylococcus
  Pneumococcus
  Anaerobic bacteria; fungi

Box 4.2 The CURB-65 scoring system

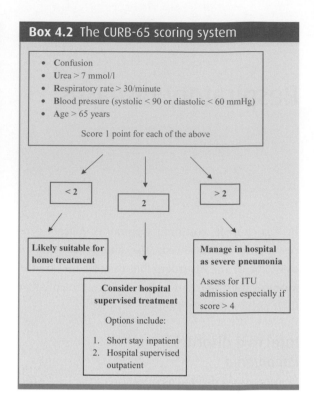

antibiotic such as clarithromycin. Gram-negative infections such as *Pseudomonas aeruginosa* are commoner as hospital-acquired infections. Guidance from the local microbiologist will guide treatment as to likely causes and their antibiotic sensitivities but treatment is often with antibiotics such as ceftazadime, gentamicin or merepenem.

Tuberculosis

Tuberculosis (TB) is a pulmonary and systemic disease caused by *Mycobacterium tuberculosis* and is spread by airborne droplet transmission. Tuberculosis is a significant worldwide problem with approximately 33% of the human population infected. The human immunodeficiency virus (HIV) epidemic has dramatically altered tuberculous epidemiology. In the UK around 5% of those with HIV are also infected with TB and only about 3% of patients with TB have HIV. However around 98% of patients with HIV are co-infected with TB in developing countries. Tuberculosis represents a complex interaction between *Mycobacterium tuberculosis* and the patient's specific immune response and non-specific resistance

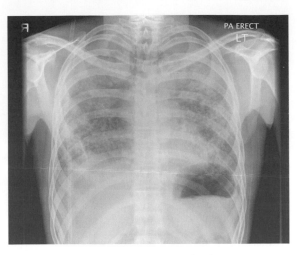

Figure 4.3 Chest X-ray in a patient with silicosis.

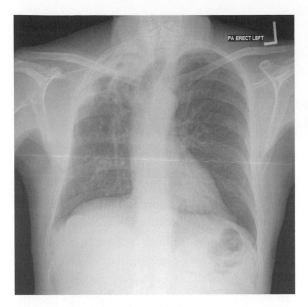

Figure 4.1 Chest X-ray demonstrating pneumonic destruction of the right upper lobe.

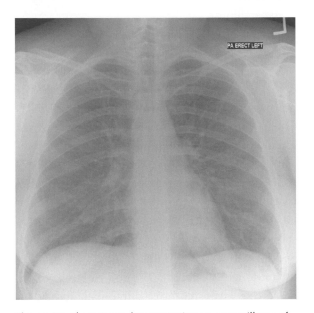

Figure 4.2 Chest X-ray demonstrating an aspergilloma of the right middle lobe.

to infection. Traditionally TB is divided into primary and post-primary TB – these descriptions being based on the characteristic evolution of TB prior to effective chemotherapy. Primary TB is the pattern of disease that is seen in a patient without specific immunity to TB. Infection is acquired by inhalation of the organism from an infected individual. The initial lesion develops in the peripheral subpleural region of the lung (Ghon focus) associated with hilar lymphadenopathy. At this stage erythema nodosum may occur. An immune response develops and healing often takes place. This stage is often asymptomatic but may leave calcified nodules on CXR. Active progression of this infection may occur with bronchial spread causing progressive consolidation and cavitation of the lung parenchyma. Lymphatic spread may cause progressive lymph node enlargement, causing bronchial compression with the development of collapse and bronchiectasis. Hematogenous spread causes generalization of the disease and can cause miliary TB and/or TB meningitis. Infection spread during this initial illness can lie dormant in any organ for years and reactivate years later. Post-primary TB is the pattern of the disease seen after the development of specific immunity. It may occur following direct progression of the initial infection or result from an endogenous reactivation of infection or from exogenous re-infection. Reactivation may occur in old age or in circumstances where immunocompetence is impaired (e.g. alcohol dependency;

immunosuppressive therapy; illness). The disease is most likely to be pulmonary, with the apices of the lungs the most common site. Clinical features tend to be non-specific and for diagnosis to be definitive the organism *Mycobacterium tuberculosis* must be identified. Once the diagnosis is suspected, repeated sputum specimens should be examined for acid- and alcohol-fast bacilli. Chest symptoms include persistent cough, sputum production and hemoptysis. Systemic symptoms may include pyrexia, sweats (particularly at night), anorexia and weight loss. Standard treatment is with 6 months of rifampicin and isoniazid supplemented by pyrazinamide and ethambutol for the first 2 months. At present drug-resistant TB is rare in initial treatments of TB but commoner in patients who have come from Africa or the Indian subcontinent or who have had previous treatment. Multidrug resistance may result from inadequate previous treatment.

Control of TB involves detection and meticulous treatment of cases of active TB, notification of the diagnosis to the public health authorities, contact tracing and targeted vaccination of groups who have a high incidence of TB. Vaccination is with BCG, a live attenuated strain of the bacillus, providing about 75% protection against TB for around 15 years. Routine vaccination of children at the age of 13 in the UK is no longer offered – rather, BCG vaccination is offered to infants in communities with a high incidence of TB and to unvaccinated individuals from countries with a high prevalence of the disease.

In addition to *Mycobacterium tuberculosis*, other mycobacteria can cause pulmonary disease. These are "atypical" or "opportunistic" mycobacteria, the commonest being *Mycoplasma kansaii, M. avium-intracellulare, M. malmoense* and *M. xenopi.* They are usually low-grade pathogens but can cause infection mainly in patients with impaired immunity or in patients with damaged lungs, e.g. in severe emphysema. They are often associated with chronic symptoms such as cough, sputum production, hemoptysis and weight loss. Treatment is often difficult and needs to be prolonged. As these organisms infect only susceptible individuals, there is no need to trace infected individuals' contacts.

Aspergillus

Aspergillus species are ubiquitous worldwide and are a rare cause of infection in healthy individuals, but in susceptible individuals these fungi can cause significant problems. The fungi are dimorphic, existing as both spores and mycelia. Following inhalation of spores from the environment, a transient saprophytic illness may occur but patients with underlying lung disease can develop persistent colonization. In the saprophytic form the organism can assume a complex pattern of mycelia growth. Depending on the susceptibility of the host, three distinct syndromes can develop:

1. Aspergilloma.
2. Allergic bronchopulmonary aspergillosis.
3. Invasive aspergillosis.

Aspergillomas can present as asymptomatic incidental findings on CXR – see Figure 4.2. They can however be associated with hemoptysis. This is usually minimal although recurrent. Findings are usually of the underlying lung disease rather than associated with the aspergilloma. The treatment is controversial. If associated with frequent or life-threatening hemoptysis, surgical resection is the treatment of choice. However, aspergillomas may spontaneously disappear in around 10% of patients and there is also a variable response to intracavity antifungal treatment. The risk of surgery may be hard to justify in the asymptomatic individual where the underlying lung disease may cause the risk of surgery to be greater than potential risks from the aspergilloma.

Allergic bronchopulmonary aspergillosis is a hypersensitivity lung disease to *Aspergillus* antigens. Patients with atopic asthma are most commonly affected and the disease has its highest incidence in individuals in their 40s. It is commonest in the UK in the winter months when the air contains the greatest quantity of *Aspergillus* spores. Clinically it presents with bronchospasm. The clinical course is characterized by cough productive of mucoid plugs, hemoptysis, intermittent febrile episodes, chest pain and recurrent pneumonia. Four major findings are suggestive of allergic bronchopulmonary aspergillosis:

1. Recurrent infiltrates on CXR.
2. Blood or sputum eosinophilia.
3. Asthma.
4. Immediate and late (6–8 hours) dermal hypersensitivity to *Aspergillus* antigens.

Treatment includes steroids, bronchodilators and sodium chromoglycate or nedocromil.

Invasive aspergillosis occurs almost exclusively in patients who are already immunocompromised, particularly those with prolonged neutropenia or on high-dose corticosteroids. It involves the lungs in 90% of cases and manifests as a necrotizing bronchopneumonia. Aggressive spread of the disease is its hallmark with metastatic spread causing endocarditis. The clinical manifestations can include dyspnea, non-productive cough, pleuritic chest pain and pyrexia.

Bronchiectasis

Bronchiectasis is usually defined as a persistent and irreversible dilatation and distortion of medium-sized bronchi. It is an acquired disease process that is not a discrete entity but rather the pathological end-stage of a variety of unrelated pulmonary infectious insults and impairment of drainage, airway obstruction or a defect in host defense (see Box 4.3). The morphological changes are usually accompanied by a chronic suppurative lung disease with cough productive of purulent sputum. Bronchiectasis may be confined to a localized area of the lung, where there is a local cause such as bronchial obstruction by a foreign body, or may be diffuse if there is a generalized cause, such as immunoglobulin deficiency.

Box 4.3 The etiology of bronchiectasis

- Severe infection
  Pertussis (whooping cough)
  Bacterial pneumonia
  Recurrent aspiration
  Tuberculosis
- Bronchial obstruction
  Foreign body
  Tumor
  Hilar lymph node adenopathy
- Cystic fibrosis
- Ciliary dysfunction
  Primary ciliary dyskinesia
  Kartagener's syndrome
- Allergic pulmonary aspergillosis
- Associated with systemic disease
  Rheumatoid arthritis
  Ulcerative colitis
- Immunodeficient states
  Hypogammaglobulinemia
- HIV infection
- Idiopathic

The main clinical feature of bronchiectasis is a chronic cough productive of copious purulent sputum. Hemoptysis is common and occasionally severe, requiring therapeutic embolization of hypertrophied bronchial arteries to control. Infective exacerbations may present with pleuritic chest pain and fever. On examination crackles may be audible over affected areas of the lungs and in more severe cases clubbing may be present. A chest X-ray may show features suggestive of bronchiectasis such as parallel tramline shadowing or cystic dilated bronchi, but it may require a high resolution CT scan to confirm diagnosis and to define extent and location of the disease process. Treatment of the specific cause is rarely possible although it is important to identify where possible what the cause is. Chest physiotherapy is the most effective method in preventing accumulation of secretion – particularly postural drainage, percussion and forced expiratory techniques. Antibiotic treatment, guided by the results of sputum microbiology, is used to suppress chronic infections and to treat exacerbations. Bronchodilator therapy may also be indicated where there is associated reversible airway obstruction. Surgical excision is a potential treatment for individuals who have a localized disease pattern and troublesome symptoms. Lung transplantation may be an option in patients who develop respiratory failure (see Chapter 14).

Lung abscess

A lung abscess is a localized collection of pus within a cavitating necrotic lesion of the lung parenchyma. It presents clinically with a history of cough with expectoration of large amounts of purulent, foul sputum and is often accompanied by hemoptysis, weight loss, pyrexia and general malaise. Drainage of pus from the abscess cavity is the main treatment. This may be achievable through bronchial drainage using postural physiotherapy. It may however be necessary to drain an abscess percutaneously by placing a drain under radiological guidance. Where medical therapy fails, surgical excision of the abscess cavity may be required.

Cystic fibrosis

Cystic fibrosis is the commonest of the potentially lethal inherited diseases in Caucasians, affecting around 1 in 2500 live births in the UK. It is inherited as an autosomal recessive disorder with 1 in 25 of the population being a carrier. Cystic fibrosis results from a mutation to a gene on the long arm of chromosome 7, which codes for a protein named cystic fibrosis transmembrane conductance regulator (CFTR). CFTR functions as a chloride channel in the membrane of epithelial cells causing reduced chloride conductance, most notably in the respiratory, gastrointestinal, pancreatic, hepatobiliary and reproductive tracts (see Box 4.4).

The dysfunction of the CFTR predisposes to severe chronic lung infections via a variety of cel-

Box 4.4 Clinical features of cystic fibrosis
• Upper airways
Sinusitis
Nasal polyps
• Lungs
Infection
Bronchiectasis
Airway obstruction
Pneumothorax
Hemoptysis
Allergic aspergillus
Respiratory failure
• Liver
Biliary cirrhosis
Hepatosplenomegaly
Portal hypertension
Gallstones
• Pancreas
Malabsorption
Malnutrition
Diabetes mellitus
• Intestines
Meconium ileus
Distal intestinal obstruction
Rectal prolapse
• Locomotor system
Arthropathy
Osteoporosis
Clubbing
• Other
Male infertility
Salty sweat

lular mechanisms. In the bronchial mucosa the reduced chloride secretion and increased sodium reabsorption results in abnormally viscous secretions, predisposing to adherence and reduced clearance of bacteria. The high salt concentrations also inactivate the lung epithelial naturally occurring antimicrobial peptides, the defensins. In addition to these defects there are also abnormal mucus glycoproteins which act as binding sites allowing bacteria to adhere to the mucosa and proliferate. As the inflammatory response is unable to clear the infection, a continuous cycle of infection and inflammation ensues. This results in progressive lung damage and bronchiectasis and ultimately respiratory failure and death. Clinical features of the respiratory component include persistent cough and purulent sputum production typical of bronchiectasis, development of digital clubbing and progressive airway obstruction with associated wheeze. Serial measurements of FEV_1 allow some monitoring of the severity and progression of disease process. Culture of sputum may initially isolate *Staphylococcus*, *Haemophilus influenza* and *Streptococcus pneumoniae*, but in older children and teenagers, isolates are likely to include mucoid strains of *Pseudomonas aeruginosa*, sometimes with pan-resistancy to antibiotic therapy. As the cycle of lung damage progresses with destruction of the lung parenchyma, increasing airway obstruction and increasing impairment of gas exchange, patients develop hypoxemia, hypercapnia and right-sided heart failure with cor pulmonale. Hemoptysis is common as the persistent inflammatory response provokes hypertrophy of the bronchial arteries. Pneumothoraces may occur, particularly in advanced disease, and may require pleurodesis if recurrent. As respiratory failure intervenes, pulmonary transplantation may be required (see Chapter 14).

Cystic fibrosis is a complex disease involving all the body's systems and therefore a multidisciplinary approach is required to the treatment of patients with the disorder. The optimal treatment is probably achieved through management at regional specialist centres. The basic elements of treatment comprise clearance of the bronchial secretions through physiotherapy; treatment of pulmonary infection by antibiotic therapy (guided by microbiological advice); correction of nutritional deficits by the use of pancreatic supplementation and dietary support; and psychological/social support for both the patient and their family.

Airway obstruction disorders
Asthma

Asthma is a disease characterized by chronic airway inflammation with increased airways responsiveness and airways obstruction. Symptoms include wheeze, dyspnea and cough. Airway obstruction is variable and may be reversible with therapy. Asthma represents a clinical syndrome that is diverse in presentation and in effects. It is multifactorial in origin but appears to arise from a combination of environmental factors and genetic susceptibility. There is a general consensus that asthma is increasing in prevalence and that this is likely to be due to environmental factors. The British Thoracic Society recommends a stepwise approach to managing asthma according to its severity (see Figure 4.4). The aim of management is to abolish symptoms, to restore normal airway function and to reduce the risk of severe life-threatening attacks. For the majority of patients the disease is controlled by a combination of a regular inhaled steroid and using an inhaled bronchodilator drug as required for symptomatic relief. The drugs used in the treatment of asthma are discussed further in Chapter 3.

ANESTHETIC CONSIDERATIONS IN ASTHMA

It is generally advisable to use an anesthetic technique that is unlikely to provoke bronchospasm. This is particularly important in thoracic anesthesia as the added airway manipulation from bronchoscopy, placement of DLT or bronchial blocker may also provoke bronchoconstriction.

Chronic obstructive pulmonary disease

Chronic obstructive pulmonary disease (COPD) is defined as a chronic slowly progressive disorder characterized by airflow obstruction. Although there is some overlap with asthma, they are different disorders with different etiologies, pathologies,

---

Step 1: Mild intermittent asthma

Inhaled short acting β–2 antagonist as required

Step 2: Regular preventor therapy

Add inhaled steroid at dose appropriate to disease severity

Step 3: Add-on therapy

Add inhaled long-acting β antagonist (LABA)

Re-assess asthma control:

- **Good response to LABA: continue**
- **Benefit from LABA but still poor control**: increase inhaled steroid dosage
- **No response to LABA**: stop LABA and increase steroid to max. dosage inhaled; if control still inadequate institute trial of other therapies, e.g. leukotriene receptor antagonist or theophylline

---

Step 4: Persistent poor control

Consider trials of :

- Increased steroid dose
- Leukotriene receptor antagonist; theophylline; β-2 antagonist tablet

---

Step 5: Continuous or frequent use of oral steroids

Use daily steroid tablet in lowest dose providing adequate control

Maintain high-dose inhaled steroid

Consider other treatments to minimize the use of steroid tablets

Refer patient for specialist care

Figure 4.4 Summary of the stepwise management of asthma in adults.

natural histories and therapy options. Whereas in asthma, airway inflammation and hyper-reactivity cause airway obstruction, in COPD alveolar destruction by emphysema causes a loss of elastic recoil and a loss of outward traction in small airways resulting in airway collapse and obstruction with air trapping and hyperinflation. COPD also encompasses chronic bronchitis due to mucus hypersecretion in the central airways and defined as cough and sputum production for 3 months of 2 successive years in a patient in whom other causes of chronic cough have been excluded. Tobacco smoking is the main cause of COPD, although only about 15% of smokers develop the disease suggesting additional factors including genetics may be important in the pathogenesis. Emphysema is thought to develop as a consequence of lung destruction by proteolytic digestion due in part to an imbalance of proteases and anti-proteases. In patients with a genetic deficiency of α_1-anti-trypsin severe emphysema develops at a young age.

ANESTHETIC CONSIDERATIONS IN COPD

Pre-oxygenation may need to be for an extended period to achieve denitrogenation. Induction and maintenance of anesthesia utilizing short-acting drugs may be preferable. The aim is to allow the patient to breathe spontaneously as soon as possible following the procedure to decrease the risks of air leakage secondary to positive pressure ventilation. Anesthesia with total intravenous technique using propofol or using a volatile such as sevoflurane may be preferred to using longer-acting agents. For muscle paralysis, drugs such as vecuronium, rocuronium or cisatracurium might be preferred for both their shorter duration of action and their absence of histamine release.

Difficulty in ventilation in COPD may occur due to airtrapping. The presence of large cystic and bullous areas may induce progressive air trapping and "pulmonary tamponade" physiology resulting in catastrophic reduction of venous return in addition to asphyxia. During ventilation it is important to monitor the volumes being delivered to and exhaled from the lungs to ensure that air is not becoming trapped.

Management of patients with emphysema is further discussed in Chapter 13.

Interstitial lung disease

Interstitial lung disease is an imprecise term referring to a diverse range of diseases which affect the alveoli and septal interstitium of the lung and which can progress to diffuse lung fibrosis. Presentation is usually with progressive dyspnea, a dry cough, lung crackles and diffuse infiltrates on chest X-ray. Lung function tests show a restrictive pattern with reduced vital capacity but a normal FEV_1/FVC ratio; a reduced transfer factor indicating impaired gas diffusion; and hypoxemia that may be accompanied initially by a relative hypocapnia. The next key investigation is usually a high-resolution CT scan as this can give an indication of the extent and pattern of the disease. Investigation should also be aimed at moving from essentially a diagnostic label of pulmonary fibrosis to a more specific diagnosis of a disease process to enable best treatment management: see Box 4.5.

Occupational lung disease

Occupational lung diseases result from the inhalation of dusts, gases, fumes or vapors encountered in the work environment. The effects of these inhaled substances vary depending on their particle size; solubility; toxicity; the duration and intensity of exposure; and the patient's susceptibility. Some substances are generally irritant in a non-specific manner or are toxic to the airways (e.g. ammonia) with all individuals exposed being similarly affected. Other substances include hypersensitivity or allergic reactions in susceptible individuals giving rise to asthma or extrinsic allergic alveolitis (see above). Asthma is the commonest form of occupational lung disease and avoidance of exposure to the inducing agent is the main form of treatment. Other substances promote fibrosis in the lung parenchyma – examples include coal dust causing coalminer's pneumoconiosis; asbestos (see Box 4.6); and silica causing silicosis (see Figure 4.3).

Patients who have suffered disability as a result of occupational lung disease will have a right to compensation from governmental agencies and they may also wish to pursue litigation against their employers. An accurate diagnosis is therefore required and these patients may present for lung biopsy. The death of a patient with a suspected occupational disease must be reported to the Coroner.

Diseases involving the pulmonary circulation
Thromboembolic disease

Pulmonary embolism usually occurs as a complication and consequence of deep vein thrombosis. These typically develop in the deep veins of the legs and then travel to the lungs causing obstruction of the pulmonary vasculature. Factors predisposing to venous thrombosis were described by Virchow as a triad of venous stasis, damage to the vein wall and hypercoagulable states. The clinical features of pulmonary embolism depend upon the size and severity of the embolism and are summarized in Box 4.7. When the diagnosis of pulmonary embolus is suspected, patients should be assessed for compatible clinical features and potential risk factors, with the exclusion of alternative diagnoses. An assay of D-dimer levels may be useful and if there remains a high clinical suspicion then definitive imaging should be performed, either with computed tomography, pulmonary angiography or ventilation/perfusion scanning. Heparin is used to achieve rapid anticoagulation and this is maintained with the use of warfarin. Where there is circulatory compromise from a massive pulmonary embolus thrombolytic therapy may be attempted. Management of chronic thromboembolic pulmonary hypertension is discussed further in Chapter 15.

Unusual forms of embolism may occur including fat (following long bone fractures); amniotic fluid peripartum; and air (usually iatrogenic).

Box 4.5 The differential diagnosis in pulmonary fibrosis

Idiopathic pulmonary fibrosis (IPF) (cryptogenic fibrosing alveolitis)

Commoner in men (M:F 2:1) and in older age groups.

Presents with progressive dyspnea, dry cough, crackles, a restrictive defect in lung function and reticulonodular infiltrates on chest X-ray.

Lung biopsy shows a typical appearance of "Usual interstitial pneumonia" with areas of interstitial fibrosis, inflammation and honeycombing.

A combination of azathioprine and steroid treatment is used but response is often poor and lung transplantation may be necessary.

Idiopathic interstitial pneumonias

- Non-specific interstitial pneumonia

  Has uniform inflammatory changes and less fibrosis on lung biopsy with ground glass opacification on CT scan.

  Responds to corticosteroids.

  Has a better prognosis than idiopathic pulmonary fibrosis.

- Cryptogenic organizing pneumonia

  Seems to be a pattern of response to various insults including amiodarone, connective tissue diseases or ulcerative colitis, but often has no identifiable cause

  Patients often present with cough, malaise, pyrexia and dyspnea with an elevated ESR

  Often responds dramatically to corticosteroids

- Desquamative interstitial pneumonia

  Relatively rare form of interstitial lung disease affecting smokers with the particular feature of alveolar macrophage desquamation

  Responds to cessation of smoking together with corticosteroids

Systemic diseases

- The typical features of IPF can occur in association with a connective tissue disease.
- These diseases may also have a number of other lung complications.
- Examples include rheumatoid arthritis; systemic sclerosis; systemic lupus erythematosus and sarcoidosis.

Inorganic dusts causing e.g. Coalminer's pneumoconiosis, silicosis and asbestosis

Organic dusts causing extrinsic allergic alveoliti

- Extrinsic allergic alveolitis is an immunologically mediated disease in which a hypersensitivity reaction occurs in a sensitized individual to an inhaled antigen. A complex immune response occurs involving antibody reactions, immune-complex formation, complement activation and cellular responses.
- Complete cessation of exposure to the provoking antigen is the main treatment.
- Examples include farmer's lung and bird-fancier's lung.

Inhaled toxins and drugs

- Paraquat.
- Amiodarone.
- Bleomycin.
- Nitrofurantoin.

> **Box 4.6** Disease conditions related to asbestos exposure
>
> - Asbestosis
>   A pneumoconiosis with diffuse parenchymal lung fibrosis resulting from prolonged heavy exposure to asbestos.
>   Presents 10–25 years after exposure with cough, progressive dyspnea, basal crackles, clubbing and a restrictive ventilator defect with impaired gas diffusion.
>   Chest X-ray shows bilateral reticulonodular shadowing.
> - Pleural plaques
>   Incidental finding on chest X-ray on workers exposed to asbestos.
>   Do not give rise to any impairment of lung function.
> - Asbestos pleurisy and pleural effusions
>   Many years after the initial exposure to asbestos, patients develop episodes of pleurisy with pleuritic pain and pleural effusions.
>   Pleural fluid is an exudate which is often blood-stained.
>   Usually spontaneously resolve but are often recurrent episodes.
> - Pleural thickening
>   When extensive causes dyspnea and a restrictive defect.
> - Asbestos-related lung cancer
>   Increased risk of lung cancer particularly in smokers.
> - Mesothelioma
>   Malignant disease of the pleura associated with a history of asbestos exposure in at least 90% of cases.
>   Average lag period of 20–40 years between exposure and development of mesothelioma.
>   Presents with pain, dyspnea, weight loss and lethargy.
>   VAT pleural biopsy may be needed to provide a definitive histopathological diagnosis.
>   Pleurodesis may control the effusion.
>   As the tumor progresses it encases the lungs and may involve the pericardium and peritoneum. Blood-borne metastases may occur.
>   Radical surgery can be attempted but has a poor success rate. Radiotherapy may shrink the tumor and often relieves symptoms of pain. Chemotherapy may also result in tumor shrinkage.
>   Poor prognosis with the majority of patients dying within 2 years.

Pulmonary hypertension

Pulmonary hypertension is a diagnosis encompassing several distinct disease processes affecting the cardiopulmonary system (see Box 4.8). It is defined as a mean pulmonary artery pressure greater than 25 mmHg at rest. The commonest setting for pulmonary hypertension in thoracic anesthesia is probably in patients who have hypoxemia secondary to chronic lung disease: WHO Class III. In this setting it may be referred to as cor pulmonale. This essentially is right ventricular hypertrophy and failure secondary to pulmonary hypertension that has arisen from secondary chronic pulmonary vasoconstriction secondary to hypoxemia.

ANESTHETIC IMPLICATIONS OF PULMONARY ARTERIAL HYPERTENSION

The pulmonary circulation is highly responsive to vasoconstrictive stimuli including vasoconstrictive drugs (e.g. metaramine, noradrenaline); hypercarbia; acidosis; agitation or pain. Increases in pulmonary arterial pressure may cause acute failure of the right ventricle with right ventricular dilatation and septal shift. This causes an acute decrease in left ventricular filling and left ventricular contractility and leads to left ventricular failure. This leads to hypotension, which in turn may lead to decreased coronary perfusion. In patients with pulmonary hypertension and right

Box 4.7 Presentations of pulmonary embolism

Massive pulmonary embolism
- Acute.
  > 50% occlusion of circulation.
  Sudden circulatory collapse with cyanosis, chest pain, hyperventilation and engorged neck veins.
  ECG may show S1, Q3, T3 pattern.
  Chest X-ray is usually unhelpful.
  Angiography shows filling defects and poor perfusion.
- Sub-acute.
  > 50% occlusion of circulation.
  Progressive severe dyspnea with no obvious cause, dyspnea even at rest.
  Raised jugular venous pressure, loud P2 on auscultation of heart.
  ECG may show RV strain pattern.
  Chest X-ray may show infarcts.
  Angiography and scan show severe perfusion defects.

Acute minor pulmonary embolism
- With infarction.
  Pleural pain, hemoptysis, effusion, fever, hyperventilation.
  Chest X-ray segmental collapse/consolidation.
- Without infarction.
  May be "silent".
  Chest X-ray and ECG may be normal.
  Angiography may show obstruction if early.
  Scan will show perfusion defects.

Chronic thromboembolic pulmonary hypertension (WHO Class IV)
- Progressive dyspnea and hyperventilation.
- May get effort syncope.
- Clinical features of pulmonary hypertension.
- ECG shows right ventricular hypertrophy and axis deviation.
- Chest X-ray may show a prominent pulmonary artery.
- Angiography may be normal or show slow circulation or peripheral pruning.
- Scan expected to show patchy irregularity.
- See Chapter 15.

Box 4.8 WHO revised classification of pulmonary arterial hypertension

Group I: Pulmonary arterial hypertension
Previously known as primary pulmonary hypertension.
Now known as idiopathic pulmonary hypertension.
Rare disease particularly affecting young women.
Treatment is specialist and may include prostacyclins such as epoprostenol and iloprost; endothelial receptor antagonists (e.g. bosentan); and selective phsophodiesterase-5-inhibitors (e.g. sildenafil). Surgical options may include atrial septostomy to decompress the failing right heart, and transplantation.

Group II: Pulmonary arterial hypertension associated with left heart disease
E.g. with chronic mitral valve disease.

Group III: Pulmonary arterial hypertension associated with lung disease and/or hypoxemia
Commonly associated with right ventricular hypertrophy and subsequent failure, known as cor pulmonale.

Group IV: Pulmonary hypertension associated with chronic thromboembolic disease
Discussed in Chapter 15.

Group V: Pulmonary arterial hypertension due to miscellaneous causes
Pulmonary hypertension can occur as a complication of collagen vascular diseases such as systemic sclerosis and systemic lupus erythematosus.
Pulmonary hypertension can also arise as a complication of drug therapy such as fenfluramine (an appetite suppressant agent).
Useful reference: Proceedings of the 3rd World symposium on pulmonary arterial hypertension, Venice, Italy. June 23–25 2003. *J Am Coll Cardiol* 2004; **43**(Suppl.12): S1–90.

ventricular hypertrophy blood flow to the right coronary ventricle assumes the diastolic phase flow dependency whereas in normal individuals the flow is both during systole and diastole. This increases susceptibility to hypotension. The response of the right ventricle is dependent on the general status of the patient – those with chronically elevated pulmonary arterial pressures have a "trained" ventricle and can often cope better with increases in pulmonary vascular resistance than those with previously normal pulmonary circulations.

Principles of management of patients with pulmonary hypertension include: identification of those at risk; invasive monitoring; maintenance of intravascular volume and myocardial contractility; and careful use of vasoactive agents. One of the most dangerous periods for these patients is at induction of anesthesia and institution of mechanical ventilation. Both the systemic vasodilation secondary to induction agents and the increase in afterload to the right heart may acutely cause decompensation of the right ventricle. Aims for anesthesia include avoiding systemic hypotension and myocardial depression; and to avoid hypoxia, hypercarbia and metabolic acidosis. The anesthetist should consider monitoring right heart function with central venous pressure and/or pulmonary arterial pressure monitoring and possibly utilize transesophageal echocardiography. Right ventricular function can be improved with inotrope and pulmonary vasodilator therapy. Management of heart failure is further discussed in Chapter 22.

Malignancy
Lung cancer

Lung cancer remains the commonest cause of cancer death worldwide. In the UK it kills about 34 000 people each year. For clinical purposes the disease is classified into two groups.

1. **Small cell carcinoma:** comprising 20% of lung cancers; also known as oat-cell carcinoma, this cancer arises from neuroendocrine cells as is evidenced by the occasional ectopic hormone production. It is highly malignant, growing rapidly and metastasizing early. Usually by the time of diagnosis it will be widely disseminated such that systemic chemotherapy is the most appropriate therapy.

2. **Non-small cell carcinoma:** comprising the remaining 80% and further divisible into **squamous-cell carcinoma** (45%); **adenocarcinoma** (20%) and **large-cell carcinoma** (15%). Adenocarcinoma has a higher incidence in patients with either localized (e.g. following TB or localized irradiation) or generalized lung fibrosis, so-called "scar carcinomas". With non-small cell carcinoma, surgical resection can offer the best opportunity for "cure" but only 10–20% of patients prove suitable for surgery. These patients require careful pre-operative assessment and staging of their disease as is discussed in Chapter 5.

Other thoracic neoplasms
Alveolar cell carcinoma

This rare tumor arises in the alveoli of the lungs and spreads along the alveolar and bronchiolar epithelium. It may be associated with the production of large amounts of mucin and copious sputum production. A transbronchial biopsy may provide diagnosis. Surgical resection is the treatment of choice if the tumor is confined to one lobe.

Carcinoid tumor

This tumor is commoner in younger patients and its occurrence is not related to smoking. It tends to be less malignant than bronchial carcinomas and is often slow growing, if locally invasive. Most arise in the main bronchi and present with hemoptysis and wheeze. Most can be cured by surgical resection. Rarely carcinoid tumor from the lung can metastasize to the liver. This may result in the secretion of substances including 5-hydroxyindolacetic acid and hence the classic "carcinoid syndrome" of flushing, wheeze and diarrhea.

Mesothelioma

This is nearly always related to asbestos exposure – see Box 4.6.

FURTHER READING

- *British Thoracic Society Guidelines for the Management of Community Acquired Pneumonia in Adults. Update 2004.* Accessed at www.brit-thoracic.org. uk
- *Tuberculosis: Clinical Diagnosis and Management of Tuberculosis and Measures for its Prevention: Clinical Guideline 33.* National Institute for Clinical Excellence 2005. Accessed at www.nice.org. uk.
- Cystic Fibrosis Trust (UK). www.cftrust.org.uk
- *British Guideline on the Management of Asthma.* British Thoracic Society/Scottish Intercollegiate Guidelines Network. Accessed at www. brit-thoracic.org.uk
- King TE. Clinical advances in the diagnosis and therapy of interstitial lung diseases. *Am J Respir Crit Care Med* 2005; **172**: 268–79.
- *The Diagnosis and Treatment of Lung Cancer: Clinical Guideline 24.* National Institute for Clinical Excellence 2005. Accessed at www.nice.org.uk.

Chapter 5

Pre-operative assessment of the thoracic surgical patient

SION BARNARD AND DOUGLAS AITCHISON

Thoracic surgery ranges from small low-risk procedures to major surgery, and for malignant and non-malignant disease. All may run into problems post-operatively. Assessment of the thoracic patient for surgery comprises two distinct areas. The first is the resectability of the lesion if malignant (or, more appropriately, correctability if benign) and the second is the fitness to withstand the morbidity it inevitably involves, referred to as operability by most surgeons. The role of pre-operative assessment in this second area is to assess the comorbidity in what is generally a relatively elderly and unfit population in order to gauge whether they will withstand the degree of surgery planned. Thorough clinical assessment coupled with appropriate further investigation is required. In assessment of resectability, radiological imaging techniques are the most commonly used methods.

When assessing malignancy, one of the major indications for thoracic surgery, it is crucial to follow the usual oncological principles of assessment. Disease must be assessed in terms of local, regional and systemic disease, with appropriate techniques used for each based on prior probabilities of disease and appropriate regional and national guidelines.

Clinical history and examination

A standard history is taken to elicit symptoms and to enable fitness for surgery (and anesthesia) to be assessed. Symptoms may include shortness of breath, chest pain and weight loss. Exercise tolerance should be assessed. A physical examination should pay particular attention to the respiratory system but also to factors that might suggest additional problems peri-operatively, for example a kyphosis. Watching a patient walk allows an informal functional assessment to be made. More formally this is part of lung function testing.

Lung function tests
Spirometry

Spirometry measures the inspiratory and expiratory volumes and more complex techniques using plethysmography also allow estimation of total lung volume. Total lung capacity (TLC) represents the lung volume at maximal inspiration. Forced vital capacity (FVC) represents the maximal exhaled volume. The forced expiratory volume (FEV) is the volume exhaled over a particular time-period. FEV over 6 seconds (FEV_6) is taken to indicate the true FVC during assessment. The forced expiratory volume over the first second (FEV_1) is a reliable

Core Topics in Thoracic Anesthesia, ed. Cait P. Searl and Sameena T. Ahmed. Published by Cambridge University Press.
© Cambridge University Press 2009.

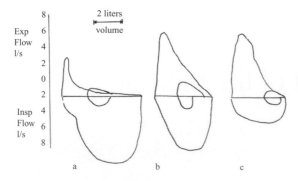

Figure 5.1 Flow volume loops.
Loop b is normal while a to the left shows small airways disease and c illustrates tracheal obstruction.

indicator of ventilatory function and is closely associated with post-operative respiratory function, discussed below. The difference between the TLC and the FVC is the residual volume (RV). This is increased in COPD and asthma.

Peak expiratory flow rate is a more reliable indicator of expiratory airflow limitation (e.g. severity of asthma for monitoring purposes) than spirometry and is measured during maximal forced expiration. Minute ventilatory volume (MVV) is the maximal volume that can be breathed over a minute. Spirometry using electronic equipment can also calculate flow-volume loops, useful for interpretation of both the inspiratory and expiratory phases. Stridor, or inspiratory obstruction, is characteristic of large airways disease i.e. of the trachea or bronchus. This is displayed by a very flattened inspiratory limb of the loop. Small airways disease, e.g. asthma, COPD, is more characteristically expressed as a flattened expiratory curve with a long tail and the appearance of an exponential type curve. These are shown in Figure 5.1.

Most of the spirometric values are normally related to height, sex and age, and equations derived from clinical series are used to predict individualized normal data. For surgical use, these are often expressed as percentage of normal predicted values to allow size-independent expression. These are important for calculations of likely post-operative respiratory function, discussed below under the BTS guidelines for lung surgery.

Gas transfer capacity

Diffusion capacity is usually measured by gas transfer factor using carbon monoxide (CO). Its high blood solubility and hemoglobin uptake is 230 times that of oxygen and practically zero concentration in atmospheric air or blood (at least in non-smokers) enable CO transfer factor ($T_L CO$) to be easily measured and independent of perfusion. Techniques rely on reasonable tidal volumes (i.e. >0.75 liters) and may be inaccurate if the patient is unable to hold a single breath. Adjustments are made for hemoglobin concentration and alveolar volume to enable normalization of values. Reference ranges for the local center are usually expressed and values may also be expressed as percentage predicted. Like spirometry, these values are important for assessment of fitness for surgery and are discussed below in the BTS guidelines for lung surgery.

Functional tests

These tests are not specific for lung function but enable a reasonably accurate assessment of the performance of combined cardiorespiratory function during exercise, provided there is no limiting musculoskeletal problem. Walking the patient down the corridor to the clinic or office is the simplest. Another is climbing flights of stairs: inability to climb more than a single flight is a very high risk indicator with any surgery; two flights without stopping is adequate for esophageal surgery; three flights as an indicator of good outcome following lobectomy; and five for pneumonectomy. Measured 6-minute walk test or numbers of shuttle runs of 10 meters between cones in 12 minutes or until stopping, are others that are more accurately measured and have been extensively validated. Measurement of the maximal oxygen uptake during exercise on a cycle or treadmill, VO_2max expressed as liters per minute or ml/kg per min for body-weight adjusted values, is the most complex but also the most closely related to fitness for surgery. A very close correlation between outcome following surgery and need for heart or lung transplantation has been shown with this test. Values below 10 ml/kg per min are insufficient for most surgical procedures. Values above 15 ml/kg per min are satisfactory for lobectomy, with several series reporting no increase in post-operative risk for any procedure with VO_2max above 20 ml/kg per min.

Arterial blood gas analysis

Measurements of arterial blood gases (ABG) allow an understanding of the carriage and delivery of oxygen, carbon dioxide and with a co-oximeter, levels of carbon monoxide or levels of met-hemoglobin containing iron in its ferric (Fe^{3+}) form that is incapable of oxygen uptake. Absolute values of pre-operative arterial carbon dioxide pressure are not directly related to outcome following surgery, with a resting hypercapnia not a contraindication to surgery, but resting hypoxia with saturations below 90% or significant desaturation on exercise are both indicators of increased operative risk.

Tremor or peripheral venous dilatation often represent hypercapnia and merit ABG analysis. Increased respiratory rate and accessory muscle use indicate underlying impairment to airflow. Arterial blood gases should also be performed on any patient cyanosed at rest, with peripheral oxygen saturation 94% or below or on oxygen therapy pre-operatively.

Radiological investigations

Initial imaging techniques involve the plain chest film, traditionally involving PA and lateral images. Sensitivity for detecting small lesions is reasonable but not as high as CT scans but the radiation exposure is very low and the investigation is widely available. Usually, localization of the lesion and approximate size estimation are possible, along with assessment of the rest of the lung fields, cardiac silhouette and the bones of the thoracic cage. More subtle signs such as presence of emphysematous bullae, pulmonary fibrosis, right-sided paratracheal lymphadenopathy (by increased tissue density adjacent to the trachea and right main bronchus which is normally adjacent to lung tissue) and loss of volume may also be observed. However, investigation is rarely limited to plain films as further information is invariably helpful for even non-surgical management.

Computerized tomography (CT)

The standard imaging technique for further chest imaging is the CT scan, usually performed to a lung cancer protocol with IV contrast and imaging at 5 mm slices from the root of the neck including the glottis down to the mid or lower abdomen to include the whole liver and spleen. An alternative technique, often used for patients with chest pain is the PE protocol in which contrast administration is timed and the scan often continued down to the lower calf. The former is more suited for thoracic surgery but the presence of tumor or thrombus within the pulmonary arteries is clearer on the latter if relevant. Computerized tomography scanning equipment is improving in sophistication and ability all the time and the newest scanners use helical multi-array sources and detectors to enable scanning of the entire chest within a single breath-hold.

The CT scan allows staging of any lung tumor, assessment for emphysema and bullous disease, shows presence of small or loculated effusions, pleural thickening and the presence of most lymph nodes above 5 mm in diameter. In addition, the tissue density often allows for a degree of diagnostic information, such as that the heavily calcified apical rounded nodule in a young patient previously exposed to TB is probably the benign remnant of a Ghon focus. Likewise, an irregularly bordered spiculated lesion with areas of differing intensity is much more likely to be malignant. Intrabronchial

Table 5.1 Lung cancer staging: 1 – TNM classification.

Tumor	Definition
T1	Tumor < 3 cm maximal dimension, surrounded by lung, or endobronchial distal to lobar bronchus
T2	Tumor > 3 cm maximal dimension, or reaching visceral pleura, or obstructive atelectasis of less than one lung, or lobar endobronchial tumor or main bronchial tumor > 2 cm from the carina
T3	Tumor involving the apex of the chest, main bronchial tumor within 2 cm of the carina, atelectasis of the entire lung, or tumor of any size invading the chest wall, parietal pleura of the mediastinum (including the phrenic nerve) or pericardium or the diaphragm
T4	Macroscopic or histological invasion of the mediastinal structures including the heart, great vessels, trachea, esophagus, carina, vertebral bodies, recurrent nerve, malignant pleural effusion, distant pleural metastases or multiple neoplastic nodules within the same lung lobe
Nodes	Definition
N0	No lymph node involvement (pN0 on pathological lymph node sampling)
N1	Metastases to hilar, interlobar, lobar or segmental nodes
N2	Metastases to ipsilateral mediastinal or subcarinal nodes
N3	Metastases to scalene or supraclavicular or contralateral nodes
Metastases	Definition
M0	No metastases
M1	Presence of metastases

lesions may also be seen on careful inspection of the lumen on several contiguous slices.

CT – tumor staging

Staging of presumed or confirmed lung cancer is performed according to strict criteria agreed internationally, as shown in Table 5.1. Tumor (T), nodal (N) and metastatic (M) levels are all assessed and classified numerically. An overall stage associated with 5-year survival can easily be read from Table 5.2.

CT – lymph nodal assessment

Lymph nodal assessment by CT must be regarded as anatomical rather than histological and is therefore not completely accurate. The absence of nodal disease is N0, presence of involved (enlarged) nodes within the lung is N1 and those within the mediastinum is N2. Contralateral, scalene or abdominal node involvement is classed as N3. In

Table 5.2 Lung cancer staging: 2 – overall staging. TNM staging presented on y and x axes, with M1 read as any T or N level within each. Approximate 5-year survivals with treatment are listed in percentages for each stage and subgroup.

TNM	N0	N1	N2	N3	M1
T1	IA 60%	IIA 34%	IIIA 13%	IIIB 3%	IV 1%
T2	IB 38%	IIB 24%	IIIA 13%	IIIB 3%	IV 1%
T3	IIB 22%	IIIA 9%	IIIA 13%	IIIB 3%	IV 1%
T4	IIIB 7%	IIIB 7%	IIIB 7%	IIIB 3%	IV 1%
M1	IV 1%	IV 1%	IV 1%	IV 1%	

the setting of lung cancer, sensitivity and specificity for involved lymph nodes range between 70–80%. Lymph nodes vary in size within the chest dependent upon age, sex and location and are generally oval in shape. Lymph node staging must be used for all enlarged nodes in patients who are potentially operable and the primary tumor resectable. Likewise, for all patients with borderline nodal size criteria or multiple small nodes in whom the primary is very advanced and/or the operability borderline, it is prudent to perform other nodal staging to prevent unnecessary non-curative surgery at greater operative risk. Further methods of lymph nodal staging include operative (mediastinoscopy and others) and functional imaging techniques such as positron emission tomography (PET), as discussed below.

CT – metastatic assessment

A computerized tomography scan is sensitive for the detection of adrenal and liver metastases from lung cancer, along with para-aortic lymphadenopathy. Ultrasound scan or PET may also be required to quantify these and differentiate from benign cysts. The presence of benign coincidental adrenalomas is a relatively common finding in the older patient and must be carefully diagnosed as it should not preclude curative lung surgery.

Although not generally recommended in the absence of neurological signs or symptoms, CT scan of the head with and without contrast is an important staging procedure in those with advanced lung tumors e.g. chest wall invasion, a possibility of lung secondaries, or with a difficulty in assessing baseline cerebral function. Presence of most cerebral metastases would prevent surgery to resect lung cancer; there is little more unfortunate than performing radical lung surgery and reconstruction only to see the patient succumb to untreatable cerebral malignancy.

Magnetic resonance imaging

Magnetic resonance imaging (MRI) scanning involves computerized reconstruction of tissue volumes from the detection of radiowaves emitted from the changes in alignment of protons within the patient lying in an intense magnetic field. There are several techniques which may be used, including the T1 and T2 relaxation times and the proton density, which all show different tissue quantification and are particularly useful for certain features. In general, however, the resolution of the MRI scan is not superior to the CT scan and it is no better at confirming the presence or absence of invasion than CT scanning. However, there are two areas where MRI scanning is routinely used in the radiological assessment of the thorax. These are both areas adjacent to bones, where CT resolution is difficult due to streak artefact from the slice reconstruction techniques used, and include assessment of Pancoast-type tumors involving the apex of the chest and brachial plexus and the neurogenic tumors of the paravertebral sulcus to assess whether there is invasion of the neural foramina or extension into the vertebral canal.

Positron emission tomography

Positron emission tomography (PET) scanning has revolutionized the imaging of the body by allowing localized measurement of tissue metabolic activity. Briefly, a radioactive isotope of fluorine is bound to deoxyglucose and administered intravenously. It is taken up as a glucose analog by metabolically active cells and only partially metabolized. It then remains stuck cytoplasmically until alternative pathways can break it down. Meanwhile the unstable fluorine isotope decays by the emission of a positron, which annihilates a nearby electron on collision with the release of two identical energy photons in opposite directions and identical constant wavelength. These are detected by a special detector array, in the newest scanners located within a CT scanner for co-localization. It is important to be aware that PET may have false negatives when metastases are present in tissues with a high underlying metabolic rate, especially brain. For this reason, scans are very rarely shown above the neck.

Table 5.3 Risks of thoracic procedures.

Procedure	Death	Bleeding	Others
Mediastinoscopy	0.3%	Sternotomy 0.1%	Pneumothorax 1% Recurrent nerve injury 1%
VAT pleural procedure	1.5%	1%	Prolonged airleak 1%
Lobectomy	2–4%	1%	Prolonged airleak 5–10%
Pneumonectomy	5–10%	1%	Bronchopleural fistula 2–10%
Lung volume reduction	5–10%	1%	Prolonged airleak 40%

Results of PET scanning are more accurate than CT scanning for nodal and metastatic assessment. A PET negative mediastinal scan is specific enough at 90–95% to rule out nodal disease in most lung cancer patients although it cannot detect micrometastases. Likewise, a positive nodal scan is indicative of increased uptake although unable to differentiate between infection or tumor metastases. Therefore, PET positive mediastinal nodes would still need further surgical assessment prior to lung resection. Despite this potential limitation, it is felt that PET scanning reduces the need for preliminary mediastinoscopy in many patients if negative and prevents a futile thoracotomy in 1 in 16 patients assessed as node-negative on CT assessment. PET scanning is proving very useful in the workup of difficult cases such as those with borderline operability, multiple metastases or extended resection, where the likelihood of disease outside the chest is higher, allowing reduction in the chance of futile surgical resection.

Operability

As discussed above, operability is generally taken to mean the ability of the patient to recover from the morbidity of the surgery. Thoracic surgical procedures range from small such as mediastinoscopy, to pneumonectomy or trauma thoracotomy which may have much higher risks. Approximate risks of death and significant complications are shown in Table 5.3.

As well as an understanding of the risks of death or major morbidity with the procedure, it is important to understand that a thoracotomy generally reduces the effective FEV_1 by around 10–15% due to pain, splinting and the mechanical effects of the incision on the chest wall musculature and ribs. The expected benefit of the surgery is also important in this context.

British Thoracic Society – Guidelines

National guidelines exist in many countries regarding the management of patients considered for lung cancer surgery. There are differences between them based mainly on the availability of advanced techniques for investigation, treatment and the precise nature of primary care, referral practice and funding. The British Thoracic Society (BTS) guidelines, published in 2001, underlie the operative management of lung cancer in the UK and a brief outline follows.

- **Age**. Risk of mortality and morbidity increases with increasing age, although acceptable rates of survival are seen in carefully selected older patients. Increased age is a significant factor increasing mortality for pneumonectomy or chest wall resection and should be considered a relative contraindication.
- **Pre-operative lung function**. Evidence from many published series shows that a pre-operative FEV_1 of over 2 liters is an indicator of low risk for pneumonectomy and

Table 5.4 Anatomical segments.					
Right lung		**Left lung**			
Upper	3	Upper	4	(proper)	2
Middle	2			(lingula)	2
Lower	5	Lower	5		
Total	10	Total	9		

pre-operative FEV_1 of over 1.5 liters is an indicator of low risk for lobectomy; in these cases, BTS guidelines do not recommend further respiratory functional testing in the absence of breathlessness.

- **Post-operative predicted lung function**, based on extrapolation from pre-operative spirometry and gas transfer, is an important predictor of surgical risk. Approximate lung function may be predicted using the normal anatomical 19 segments and the estimated number to be resected, using the following formula:

$$ppoFEV_1 = FEV_1 * (19 - R)/19$$

where R is the proposed number of segments in the resection and $ppoFEV_1$ is the post-operative predicted FEV_1.

The same formula may be used to calculate the predicted gas transfer value.

The numbers of segments in each lobe are listed in Table 5.4. Evidence from many published series shows that a post-operative predicted $FEV_1 > 40\%$ and post-operative predicted $T_LCO > 40\%$ of normally predicted with no desaturation is sufficient for acceptable operative risk. An absolute lower limit of FEV_1 of 800 ml is recommended. If there is significant pathology affecting the lung to be resected, it may be that the above formula will underestimate the predicted post-operative lung function. In the setting of segmental or lobar collapse of the affected lung, the number of affected segments should be subtracted from the numerator and the denominator of the above equation. If the results are borderline or there is doubt about the function following resection, the differential perfusion from radionuclide studies is invaluable. If patients have both post-operative predicted FEV_1 and T_LCO below 40%, the patients are high-risk and should be considered for radiotherapy, chemotherapy or very limited (e.g. wedge) resection. All other patients should be considered intermediate risk and should undergo exercise testing with shuttle runs or VO_2max. Fewer than 25 shuttles or below 15 ml/kg per min oxygen uptake are indicators of very high surgical risk. Above these values, risks may be acceptable.

- **Cardiac assessment**. All patients undergoing lung resection should have resting 12-lead electrocardiography and echocardiography in the presence of cardiac murmur or known valvular or structural heart disease. No patient should undergo surgery within 6 weeks of myocardial infarction (MI) and all patients within 6 months of MI should have a cardiology opinion. Previous coronary artery bypass grafts should not limit surgery if the patient has adequate functional capacity and is asymptomatic. Patients with a single risk factor for coronary disease but no symptoms are at low risk and do not need further investigation. Those with previous disease but adequate functional capacity, e.g. able to climb a single flight of stairs comfortably likewise do not need further investigation. Those at high risk should undergo exercise or other stress testing and consideration of percutaneous or surgical intervention prior to lung surgery as appropriate.

- **Assessment of other organ systems**. Patients should have adequate nutritional status: weight more than 10% below ideal or low serum albumen levels should be taken as indicators of increased or high surgical risk. Liver function testing should also be performed to highlight evidence of dysfunction or indication of metastatic disease.

- **Renal function**. Renal impairment is an indicator of increased risk for major surgery but should not necessarily contraindicate potentially curative surgery. Renal dialysis should prompt careful consideration of the expected survival with and without malignancy but likewise should not contraindicate lower risk potentially curative procedures.
- **Brain**. In patients of intermediate or higher risks with surgery, extended staging may include head CT scanning to exclude metastasis (as mentioned in the imaging section). Careful consideration of those with progressive cerebral disease such as dementia, Parkinson's or ischemic strokes should be made as both increased peri-operative risk and reduced long-term survival will result.
- **Blood**. Blood testing should exclude the presence of untreated anemia. Polycythemia is common in heavy smokers and those with lung disease and is an increased risk factor for thrombo-embolic complications peri-operatively. Presence of myelodysplastic syndromes has similar effects along with an increased risk of hemorrhage and is associated with poorer long-term survival although some patients with low-grade forms may have a reasonable prognosis. The presence of hypnoatremia suggests the syndrome of inappropriate ADH secretion (SIADH).

FURTHER READING

- British Thoracic Society and Society of Cardiothoracic Surgeons of Great Britain and Ireland Working Party. Guidelines on the selection of patients with lung cancer for surgery. *Thorax* 2001; **56**: 89–108.
- Mountain CF, Libstitz HI, Hermes KE. *A Handbook for Staging, Imaging and Lymph Node Classification*. Charles P. Young, 2003.
- Strand TE, Rostad H, Moller B, *et al*. Risk factors for 30-day mortality after resection of lung cancer and prediction of their magnitude. *Thorax* 2007; **62**: 991.

Chapter 6

Lung isolation

DAVID PLACE

With the developments in thoracoscopic and minimally invasive cardiac surgery, the absolute indications for lung isolation have expanded. These developments have coincided with the availability of new bronchial blocker devices. These devices may have advantages over the traditional double lumen endobronchial tube (DLT) in specific circumstances.

This chapter aims to give an overview of the indications and techniques available for lung isolation in adult patients, using devices currently available in the UK.

History

Before the development of the Carlens left-sided DLT in 1950, a tube that was designed for differential lung spirometry, anesthetists used either single lumen tubes or bronchial blockers to produce lung isolation. The major developments in devices are listed in Table 6.1.

Current single-use plastic DLTs are based on the Robertshaw design; a red rubber tube, oval in cross-section with two D-shaped lumens placed laterally to each other to maximize internal luminal size and reduce gas flow resistance. The right-sided version has a right upper lobe ventilation slot in the bronchial portion of the tube. The bronchial and tracheal cuffs of plastic DLTs have high volume,

low pressure cuffs, in order to reduce the risk of mucosal trauma.

In the 1980s, the Univent tube, a combined single lumen tube with incorporated bronchial blocker, became available. This was further revised recently to become the Univent torque control blocker (TCB) (Vitaid Ltd.), the changes enabling improved control of the bronchial blocker.

Today, the availability of the fiberoptic bronchoscope (FOB) has encouraged the use and development of bronchial blockers which would previously have required rigid bronchoscopy for placement. Over the past decade several independent bronchial blockers have been developed which can be positioned under FOB guidance, and used in conjunction with standard single lumen tracheal tubes. Other balloon-tipped catheters, such as Fogarty embolectomy catheters, have also been used as bronchial blockers.

Indications for lung isolation

Two broad categories encompass the main reasons to perform lung isolation:

1. To prevent contamination of normal lung with blood or pus.
2. To control the distribution of ventilation. This can be to facilitate surgical exposure or to enable ventilation in cases of airway disruption,

Table 6.1 Major developments in lung isolation devices.

Date	Name	Device type
1932	Gale & Waters	Endobronchial tube with carinal cuff
1936	Magill	Right and left endobronchial tubes with short cuffs
1936	Magill	Red rubber endobronchial blocker
1950	Carlens	Left-sided DLT, carinal hook. Oval in horizontal plane
1955	Macintosh & Leatherdale	Left endobronchial tube, tracheal and bronchial cuffs, tracheal suction channel
1955	Macintosh & Leatherdale	Cuffed tracheal tube with left bronchus blocker and bronchial suction channel, Curved to enable blind insertion
1957	Green & Gordon	Right endobronchial tube, carinal hook and upper lobe ventilation slot. Bronchial and tracheal cuffs
1960	Bryce–Smith & Salt (left-sided version 1959 Bryce-Smith)	Right DLT, oval in anterior–posterior plane, slit in endobronchial cuff for upper lobe ventilation
1962	Robertshaw	Right and left sided DLTs Oval cross-section in lateral plane, no carinal hooks, right upper lobe ventilation slot. Increased inner luminal diameters
1982	Univent tube (Vitaid Ltd.)	Univent tube; combined single lumen tube and retractable bronchial blocker
1999	Arndt blocker (Cook)	Wire guided bronchial blocker. High volume low pressure cuff. Coupled with fiberoptic bronchoscope via a monofilament loop during insertion
2003	Cohen Flexitip Endobronchial blocker (Cook)	Flextip bronchial blocker. Tip flexed under control from wheel at hub. Positioned under FOB guidance. Used with standard tracheal tube

(Modified from Pappin JC. The current practice of endobronchial intubation. *Anaesth* 1979; **34**: 57–64.)

Table 6.2 Absolute indications for lung isolation.

To prevent contamination of normal lung
  Major pulmonary hemorrhage
  Bronchopleural fistula with empyema
  Lung abscess
  Whole lung lavage for alveolar proteinosis (rare)

To control the distribution of ventilation
  Bronchopleural fistula
  Traumatic airway disruption
  Giant bullae at risk of rupture

Allow surgical access
  Thoracoscopic surgery
  Minimally invasive cardiac surgery

airway fistulae, giant bullae or other severe unilateral lung disease. Table 6.2 lists examples of absolute indications for lung isolation.

In current clinical practice, most surgeons would expect lung isolation to facilitate surgical access for the majority of procedures requiring thoracotomy. It is an absolute requirement for thoracoscopic surgery and many procedures are now performed using video-assisted thoracoscopy (VATS).

Other procedures that usually require lung isolation include esophageal surgery, surgery of descending thoracic aorta, spinal surgery via thoracotomy and chest wall resection.

Methods and choice of technique

The DLT, bronchial blocker and an appropriately sized single lumen tracheal tube can all produce lung isolation, if placed in a main stem bronchus. No one technique has overarching advantages for all situations, but each lends itself to certain clinical applications. The choice will be influenced by the anesthetist's experience, certain patient factors such as abnormal airway anatomy, and surgical requirements.

The double lumen endobronchial tube

Double lumen endobronchial tubes in common use are plastic, oval in cross-section and have an antero-posterior curve corresponding to the oropharyngeal curve and a right or left lateral

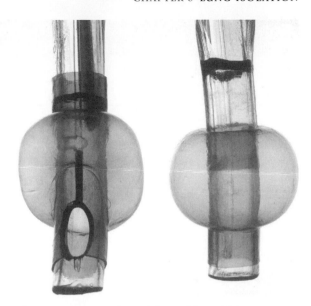

Figure 6.2 A comparison of the endobronchial components of right and left Mallinckrodt bronchocaths.

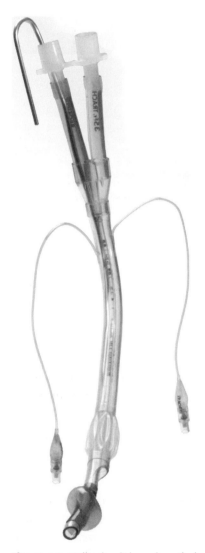

Figure 6.1 Mallinckrodt bronchocath double lumen endobronchial tube (right) (DLT).

curve corresponding to tracheobronchial anatomy (Figure 6.1). One lumen opens in the trachea below the tracheal cuff and the other terminates at the tip of the endobronchial portion. On right-sided tubes there is an endobronchial ventilation slot to allow ventilation of the right upper lobe (RUL) (Figure 6.2). The arrangement of the cuff and slot varies depending on tube manufacturer. The endobronchial cuff is colored blue to assist with identification during bronchoscopy.

The main advantages of the DLT over other methods are:

1. Rapid inflation and deflation of either lung without repositioning.
2. Suction and fiberoptic inspection to either lung is immediately possible.

Due to their larger size, DLTs are more difficult to insert than single lumen tubes, particularly if laryngoscopy is difficult. Table 6.3 compares the internal and external dimensions of DLTs and single lumen tubes. They are unsuitable for prolonged weaning from ventilation due to higher airflow resistance and patient discomfort from the bulkier tube.

Table 6.3 A comparison of the approximate outer diameters (OD) of single lumen and double lumen tubes of different sizes (actual sizes vary between manufacturers).

Single lumen tube		Double lumen tube	
Inner diameter (mm)	OD (mm)	size (Ch)	OD (mm)
7	9.5	32	10.7
7.5	10.2	35	11.7
8	10.8	37	12.3
8.5	11.4	39	13
9	12.1	41	13.7

When using the double lumen tube, there are two important considerations:

1. Choice of tube side; right or left?
2. Which size of tube to use?

Right or left-sided tube?

The right main bronchus is much shorter than the left; 2 cm rather than approximately 5 cm on the left. The position of the right upper lobe take off is also variable and can even arise from the trachea. For these reasons it may be difficult, or impossible, to simultaneously isolate the right lung and ventilate the right upper lobe using a right-sided DLT. Even with correct initial placement, minimal movement of the tube may result in failure to ventilate the right upper lobe. This can result in hypoxia during one-lung ventilation and may predispose to post-operative right upper lobe collapse.

As the left main bronchus is longer, it does not present the same problems. Left endobronchial intubation usually provides a safe and stable tube position, and is the preferred technique, unless there is an absolute indication for a right DLT (Table 6.4). The greater angulation of the left main bronchus may occasionally create technical difficulties with endobronchial intubation.

Tube sizing

Plastic DLTs are available in Charriere (Ch) gauge (or French gauge (F)) sizes 26, 28, 32, 35, 37, 39 and

Table 6.4 The indications for a right-sided double lumen endobronchial tube.

Left pneumonectomy*
Left lung transplantation
Intraluminal tumor or stent in left main bronchus
External compression of left main bronchus
Left tracheobronchial disruption
Acute angulation of left main bronchus

* Left-sided tube can be used with surgical cooperation.

41 although not all manufacturers produce their tubes in all of these sizes. Most anesthetists choose the size of tube based on the patient's height and sex (Table 6.5), although a more accurate approach may be to take measurements of tracheobronchial dimensions from scans and X-rays. A correctly sized tube should pass easily through the glottis and the endobronchial component should enter the bronchus without resistance. If the tube is under-sized it may be advanced too far into the distal airways, resulting in obstruction of lobar bronchi and risk of barotrauma and volutrauma to ventilated segments.

It has been shown by Brodsky *et al.* that tracheal width, measured at the level of the clavicles on PA chest X-ray, could predict left DLT size (Table 6.6). This has not been successfully applied in all patient populations.

Table 6.5 A guide to left double lumen endobronchial tube (DLT) size based on patients height and sex.

Women		Men	
Height (m)	Left DLT size (Ch)	Height (m)	Left DLT size (Ch)
< 1.5	32	< 1.6	37
1.5–1.6	35	1.6–1.7	39
> 1.6	37	> 1.7	41

Table 6.6 Suggested left double lumen endobronchial tube (DLT) size according to tracheal width measured on PA chest X-ray at level of clavicles.

Measured tracheal width (mm)	Left DLT size (Ch)
= 18	41
= 16	39
= 15	37
= 14	35
= 12.5	32

(From Brodsky JB, Macario A, Mark JBD. Tracheal diameter predicts double-lumen tube size: a method for selecting left double-lumen tubes. *Anesth Analg* 1996; **82**: 861–4.)

Pre-operative chest X-rays and scans should be carefully examined to assess tracheobronchial anatomy. Distortion, angulation or compression of major airways may influence choice of lung isolation technique.

Insertion of the DLT

The tube is supplied with a wire stylet placed in the bronchial lumen to increase rigidity. This should be in place prior to insertion. Laryngoscopy is performed in the usual way and the tip of the tube is passed through the vocal cords with the endobronchial tip pointing anteriorly. After passage through the cords the wire stylet should be removed before further tube advancement. The tube is then advanced and rotated 90° either to the left or right depending on which bronchus is to be intubated. Advancement of the tube is stopped on sensation of slight resistance. Alternatively, the tube can be inserted to a predetermined depth using the guide for left-sided tubes; 29 cm at the incisor teeth for a patient 170 cm tall, ± 1 cm for every ± 10 cm of height.

The FOB can also be used at the outset to position the tube by advancing the tube over the FOB into the appropriate bronchus. This may be particularly useful in patients of short stature where the trachea will be short, or where difficult positioning is predicted due to tracheobronchial anatomy.

The tracheal cuff is then inflated and ventilation is commenced through both lumens. Care should be taken with these initial inflations as it is possible to deliver the entire tidal volume to a single lobe if an undersized tube has passed beyond a bronchial division during blind insertion.

Checking DLT position

Traditionally tube position has been assessed using auscultation (Table 6.7), but with the advent of fiberoptic bronchoscopy, high rates of malposition were discovered despite satisfactory findings at auscultation. Blind placement of right-sided disposable plastic tubes has a high incidence of right upper lobe obstruction and so FOB assessment of right DLTs is now considered mandatory. An important landmark is the trifurcation of the RUL bronchus which should be visible using the FOB through the ventilation slot of a correctly positioned tube

Table 6.7 A method to check double lumen endobronchial tube position using chest auscultation.

1. Ventilate through both lumens whilst inflating tracheal cuff to abolish air leak, and ensure equal air entry in all lung fields

2. Clamp connector to tracheal lumen and open tracheal lumen to air

3. Ventilate through bronchial lumen whilst slowly inflating bronchial cuff until air leak from open tracheal lumen abolished*

4. Auscultate chest to ensure the intended lung is isolated

5. Clamp bronchial connector and open bronchial lumen to air

6. Ventilate through tracheal lumen only and auscultate to ensure air entry to non-intubated lung only

* Should only require small volume of air (< 3 ml) to seal endobronchial cuff with optimal tube size.

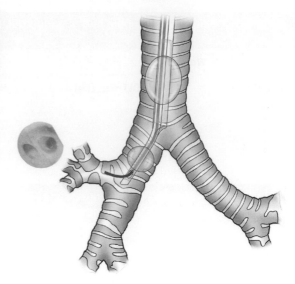

Figure 6.3 A diagram showing a correctly positioned right double lumen endobronchial tube (DLT). The fiberoptic bronchoscope view of the trifurcation of the right upper lobe is shown.

(Figure 6.3). The FOB should be passed through both lumens of the DLT to ensure that lobar bronchi are patent and that the position at the carina is correct. The proximal edge of the bronchial cuff should be just visible beyond the carina and not herniating above it.

The endobronchial cuff should be inflated with the minimal amount of air to produce a seal, in order to avoid high cuff pressures which may lead to mucosal damage. Tube position should be rechecked with any change in patient position. Moving from supine to lateral decubitus frequently results in movement of the tube, usually in a cephalad direction.

Complications of DLT insertion

Minor upper airway trauma, dental damage and failed intubation are potential complications occurring with the use of any device used to intubate the trachea. Malposition resulting in failure to produce lung isolation, airway obstruction, hypoxemia and atelectasis can occur with the use of the DLT. Rarer complications include tracheal or bronchial rupture and even incorporation of the device into a surgical staple line. Care during insertion, removal of the wire stylet before tube advancement and caution with endobronchial cuff inflation may reduce the risk of serious complications.

Bronchial blockers

There are two main configurations of bronchial blockers.

1. The blocker is incorporated into a channel in the wall of a tracheal tube as in Univent TCB (Vitaid Ltd.) (Figures 6.4 and 6.5).

2. Independent catheter as in Arndt Blocker (Cook) (Figure 6.6), Cohen Flextip Endobronchial Blocker (Cook), Uniblocker (Vitaid Ltd.), Coopdech blocker (Smiths Medical).

All of the specifically designed bronchial blockers are balloon-tipped catheters with a central channel to allow suction, lung deflation and insufflation of

nal diameter is larger than standard single lumen tracheal tubes with the same internal diameter. The tube can be used as a standard single lumen tracheal tube until lung isolation is required, at which time the blocker is advanced into the required position in either main bronchus under vision via FOB. To assist with placement, the tracheal tube can be rotated towards either left or right main bronchus as appropriate.

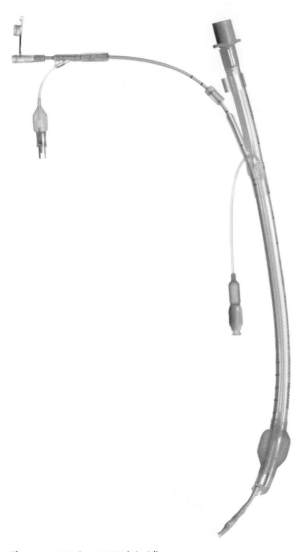

Figure 6.4 Univent TCB (Vitaid).

oxygen. They differ in their method of manipulation of the catheter tip during placement.

The Univent TCB is unique in that it combines a single lumen silicone tracheal tube with a retractable 2 mm diameter endobronchial blocker incorporated into the anterior wall of the tube. The cuff of the blocker is low pressure high volume and requires approximately 2–8 ml of air to seal, depending on the size of the airway to be occluded. An increasing range of sizes are available, including pediatric, but it is important to realize that the exter-

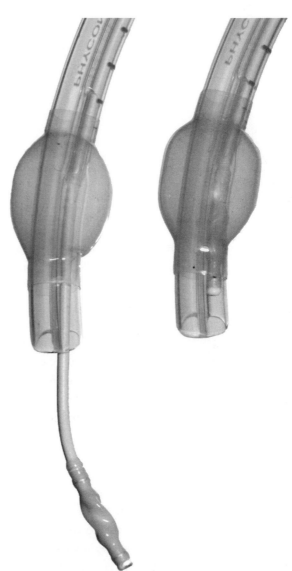

Figure 6.5 Tip of Univent TCB (Vitaid) showing tracheal cuff and blocker extended and retracted.

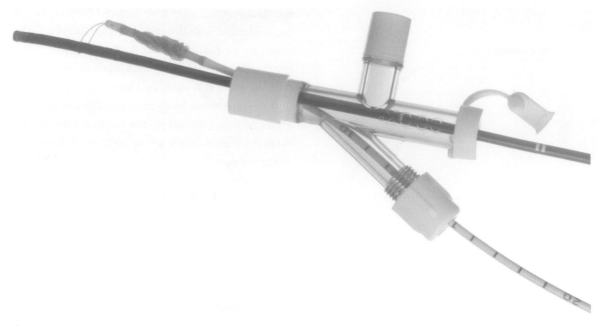

Figure 6.6 Arndt wire guided endobronchial blocker coupled to fiberoptic bronchoscope via the three-way multiport adaptor.

The independent bronchial blocker catheters can all be positioned coaxially down a standard tracheal tube under FOB guidance. A three-way, multiport adaptor allows insertion of blocker and bronchoscope without interrupting ventilation of the patient. The Arndt wire guided endobronchial blocker (Cook) is coupled to the FOB via a monofilament loop protruding from the distal end of the central channel, allowing the blocker to be guided directly into the required bronchus (Figure 6.6). The guide wire loop should be withdrawn for the central channel to allow egress of air, lung deflation and enable suction of secretions. Oxygen can be insufflated if required. The loop can be reinserted to allow repositioning of the blocker. The Cohen Flextip blocker is not directly coupled to the scope but it can be positioned under vision during FOB by a combination of catheter rotation and by flexing the tip which is controlled by a wheel at the proximal end of the catheter. This allows repositioning at any time during its use. The Uniblocker and Coopdech catheters both have a slightly flexed tip which enables the blocker to be directed to either main bronchus with a combination of advancement and rotation of the catheter under vision via FOB.

The Arndt blocker catheter is available in two sizes; 5F and 9F with corresponding minimum recommended tracheal tube sizes of 4.5 mm and 7.5 mm respectively. A pediatric bronchoscope is required and the FOB and catheter should be lubricated prior to insertion to facilitate passage through the tracheal tube.

The Cohen Flextip catheter is currently available in size 9F only.

Complications associated with the use of bronchial blockers

Complications with the use of bronchial blockers include malposition and displacement resulting in life-threatening airway obstruction and hypoxia.

Failure to clear secretions through the small central channel of a bronchial blocker resulting in

Table 6.8 Comparison of lung isolation techniques.

Double lumen tubes	Independent bronchial blockers	Univent torque control blocker (TCB)
Advantages	**Advantages**	**Advantages**
Rapid inflation and deflation of either lung	Difficult airway (can be used with single lumen tracheal tube)	Difficult airway (although bulkier than equivalent single lumen tracheal tube)
FOB inspection and suction to either lung possible	Patients already intubated	Tube change not required for post-operative ventilation
Stable position (Left)	Tube change not required for post-operative ventilation	Lobar collapse possible
	Lobar collapse possible	
Disadvantages	**Disadvantages**	**Disadvantages**
Difficult to place in difficult airway	FOB required for placement	Tube change required if patient already ventilated
Tube change required if patient already ventilated	Slow lung deflation	FOB required for blocker placement
Unsuitable for prolonged post-operative ventilation	Small channel for suction	Small suction channel
	Repositioning required for sequential lung collapse	Blocker needs repositioning for sequential lung collapse

soiling of normal lung after cuff deflation has been reported.

Which device to use? (Table 6.8)

Studies have shown that the DLT, independent bronchial blocker and Univent tube can all produce lung isolation and satisfactory operating conditions. In one study by Campos *et al.* the incidence of failure to position the device correctly by infrequent thoracic anesthetists was similar for all three methods. Lung deflation tends to be slower with BB devices whereas the DLT gives unrestricted access to both lungs for suction, bronchoscopy and insufflation.

However, BB devices have a role in the management of patients requiring lung isolation who are already intubated or who require post-operative ventilation, where exchanging tubes may be hazardous. They may also be specifically indicated where lobar blockade (Figure 6.7) is required. This may be required in patients who have undergone previous lung resection and are undergoing further thoracic surgery.

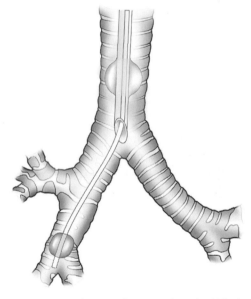

Figure 6.7 A diagram showing a bronchial blocker placed in the right bronchus intermedius enabling blockade of just the middle and lower lobes.

Lung separation and the difficult airway

Because of the size and shape of DLTs, orotracheal intubation can be difficult in situations where

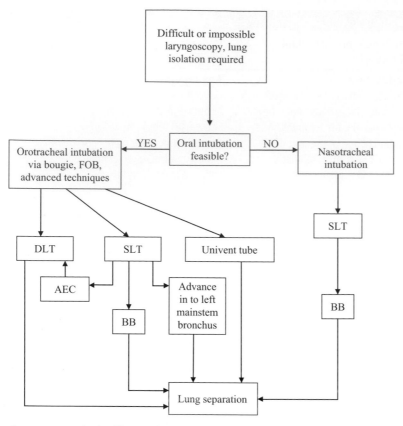

Figure 6.8 Methods of lung isolation in the patient with difficult laryngoscopy. AEC, airway exchange catheter; BB, bronchial blocker; SLT, single lumen tube; DLT, double lumen tube; FOB, fiberoptic bronchoscope.

intubation with a single lumen tube can be performed with ease. This problem is greatly amplified in patients with difficult laryngoscopy. Awake fiberoptic intubation with a DLT has been reported, but it is likely to be technically challenging. An alternative is to secure the airway with a single lumen tube and then proceed with bronchial blockade or change to a DLT using an airway exchange catheter. Figure 6.8 outlines some of the possibilities for airway management in a patient with difficult laryngoscopy. Where airway exchange catheters are being employed it is essential to ensure the free passage of the catheter inside the bronchial lumen of the DLT before proceeding.

Alternative laryngoscopes have been employed with success in patients with difficult laryngoscopy and the surgeon may be able to pass a bougie or

airway exchange catheter into the trachea during rigid bronchoscopy.

Patients with tracheostomy

Single lumen tracheal tubes, standard DLTs and bronchial blockers have all been used to provide lung isolation in patients with tracheostomy. Rusch manufacture right- and left-sided DLTs for use through a tracheostomy. These tubes are shorter and appropriately curved compared with standard DLTs and are appropriate for longer-term ventilation where lung isolation is required. The choice of other techniques will be governed by the size of the tracheostomy stoma and the reason for lung isolation. The availability of bronchial blockers has simplified the management of these patients.

Key points

- The left-sided DLT remains the device of choice for the majority of procedures requiring lung isolation in adult patients.
- Familiarity with the bronchoscopic appearance of tracheobronchial anatomy is essential for the safe and effective placement of devices for lung isolation.
- The position of the right upper lobe bronchus can prevent correct placement of the right-sided DLT and prevent complete right lung isolation by a single bronchial blocker.
- Bronchial blockers have a key role in providing lung isolation in patients with a difficult airway, those requiring post-operative ventilation and those already intubated and receiving critical care.
- The free passage of bougies, airway exchange catheters, bronchial blockers and bronchoscopes through the intended tracheal tube should be established before proceeding with clinical intervention.

FURTHER READING

- Arndt GA, Buchika S, Kranner PW *et al.* Wire-guided endobronchial blockade in a patient with a limited mouth opening. *Can J Anaesth* 1999; **46**: 87–9.

- Brodsky JB, Lemmens HJM. Left double-lumen tubes: clinical experience with 1,170 patients. *J Cardiothorac Vasc Anesth* 2003; **17**: 289–98.
- Brodsky JB, Macario A, Mark JBD. Tracheal diameter predicts double-lumen tube size: a method for selecting left double-lumen tubes. *Anesth Analg* 1996; **82**: 861–4.
- Campos JH. Current techniques for perioperative lung isolation in adults. *Anesthesiology* 2002; **97**: 1295–1301.
- Campos JH, Hallam EA, Van Natta T, Kernstine KH. Devices for lung isolation used by anaesthesiologists with limited thoracic experience: Comparison of double lumen endotracheal tube, Univent ® Torque Control Blocker, and Arndt Wire-guided endobronchial blocker ®. *Anesthesiology* 2006; **104(2)**: 261–6.
- Cohen E. Methods of lung separation. *Curr Opin Anaesthesiol* 2002; **15**: 69–78.
- Fitzmaurice BG, Brodsky JB. Airway rupture with double lumen tubes. *J Cardiothorac Vasc Anesth* 1999; **13**: 322–9.
- Hanallah MS, Benumof JL, Ruttiman UE. The relationship between left mainstem bronchial diameter and patient size. *J Cardiothorac Vasc Anesth* 1995; **9**: 119–21.
- Mirzabeigi E, Johnson C, Ternian A. One-lung anesthesia update. *Semin Cardiothorac Vasc Anesth* 2005; **9(3)**: 213–26.

Chapter 7

Management of one-lung ventilation

LEENA PARDESHI AND IAN CONACHER

Physiologically, on the institution of one-lung ventilation (OLV), the patient, by continuing to perfuse a non-ventilated lung, is positioned on the steep part of the oxygen dissociation curve: what has been described as analogous to *in the mountaineer "death zone."* Unlike the latter the inhalation of high concentrations of oxygen may not avert disaster. One-lung ventilation is never safe. It is this simple fact that makes attention to detail vital. The double lumen endobronchial tube (DLT) sited "too far," or the inadequately ventilated dependent lung adds the few critical degrees to the percentage of the cardiac output that is desaturated to take the situation beyond one salvageable with high inspired oxygen.

Notwithstanding interference of anesthetic agents with natural controls in matching of ventilation/perfusion, and of an open pneumothorax and lateral decubitus position compromising pulmonary and cardiovascular physiology, in practice, all problems of gas exchange should be seen as reflecting the conduct of OLV, and correctable by safe anesthetic or surgical maneuvre.

Fundamentals of fractional inspired oxygen (FiO$_2$)

There is a paradox with using fractional inspired oxygen (FiO$_2$) 1.0. If necessary, then almost by definition there is a problem. Safe-enough oper-

ating conditions for pulmonary *resection* can be achieved with less, providing criteria for defining fitness have been met and by attention to detail in the conduct of OLV. This is not a statement of a cavalier attitude with the requirement for 100% oxygen or for its use in those already close to respiratory failure who may have to undergo OLV to facilitate a diagnostic or therapeutic process. Automatic use remains paramount as a therapeutic and first aid measure. Requirement is, however, to be read as a clinical signal of a treatable OLV problem (see Table 7.1).

Planning OLV

An expectant attitude is required, with some sense of those who may not cope with anything other than perfect lung separation and in whom a default position of recruiting the "surgeon's' lung" may be necessary. As a working guide, those with a predicted FEV$_1$ > 40% pre-operative values should pass through an OLV process without too much difficulty and few problems. Those with a predicted FEV$_1$ < 40% may well require support including post-operative ventilation. Planning, prediction and preparedness for improvisation are important: the former essential for guiding the process, and the latter for dealing with the unexpected. These define the level of monitoring required, early and direction of interventions, intra-operative conduct and

Core Topics in Thoracic Anesthesia, ed. Cait P. Searl and Sameena T. Ahmed. Published by Cambridge University Press.
© Cambridge University Press 2009.

Table 7.1 First aid.

1. Increase (if not already done) the FiO_2 to 1.0
2. Go to manual IPPV. Request surgeon to stop operating
3. Aspirate for secretions etc. ventilated lung
4. If desaturation continues recruit surgeon's lung
5. Once patient safely oxygenated, define problem, adjust and resolve situation (see below for diagnoses and options)
6. Invite the surgeon to continue

Table 7.2 Operation groups as guide to level of care.

Group 1	Group 2
Pulmonary resection	Pneumonectomy
Lobectomy	Chest wall resection
Wedge resection	Lung volume reduction surgery
Open thoracotomy	Lung transplantation
Lung biopsy	Esophagectomy
Thoracoscopic	
Lung biopsy	
Pleurodesis	
Sympathectomy	
Thymectomy	

Table 7.3 A checklist of immediately available equipment.

Stethoscopes

Standard endotracheal tubes

Lung separators: both right- and left-sided*

Rigid bronchoscope

Fiberoptic bronchoscope

Bougies and airway exchangers

Regional analgesia equipment and drugs – paravertebral and epidural

* For women: 35, 37, and 39 Fr. For men: 37, 39 and 41 Fr. In general the largest tube that will fit should be tried. This decreases the airway resistance and makes fiberoptic examination easier.

the post-operative management. A pleural operation in an ASA I patient, or a lobectomy in an ASA II patient, for instance, needs a level that is similar to that required by a patient undergoing a relatively minor abdominal operation (see Table 7.2, Group 1). Whereas, for the pneumonectomy, complicated lobectomy or esophagectomy, the level required is that of the patient undergoing cardiopulmonary bypass (Group 2). In the event of problems arising, e.g. hemorrhage, shift from lobectomy to pneumonectomy, prolonged OLV or lung handling (< 90 min) then Group 1 category should be assigned to the Group 2 level of intervention,

care and management. Theoretically, it should not matter whether the surgical approach is via a lateral thoracotomy or thoracoscopy, but in practice when surgical access is restricted, the options for keeping the lung collapsed and out of the operating field are more limited.

Preparation for OLV in the anesthetic room

The institution of OLV can be problematic in approximately 20% of any case mix. A significant number will prove difficult at the lung separator insertion stage. The usual conditions of difficult intubation pertain, as well as some specific to the thoracic discipline and the pathologies encountered and exacerbated by the structure and bulk of some lung separators. The checklist in Table 7.3 is designed to cover the consistently and historically described difficulty posed in securing left lung isolation. The choice of lung separator has been discussed in Chapter 5.

Choice of anesthetic technique

There is now little place for nitrous oxide as a carrier gas in thoracic practice: air–oxygen mixes are the routine. A dominant theme for 40 years has been the influence of general anesthetics on hypoxic pulmonary vasoconstriction (HPV) (see also Chapter 2). Although recognized as a potential problem, modern perspectives and evidence suggest that importance is over-rated and distracts from more likely reasons for changes in the shunt fraction. These are in practice more mechanical than biological: the effect of an open pneumothorax, collapse of lung and gravity on assumption of the decubitus position all in some measure favor flow to ventilated areas. It remains to be reinforced that the phenomenon of HPV is scientifically interesting but should never be invoked to justify poor technique or use of the hypothetical in the clinical arena. There is now little difference when modern volatile agents or total intravenous anesthesia are used, suggesting that the effects of techniques using nitrous oxide and/or potent cardiac depressants such as halothane may have been confounders in some of the early studies. As a general rule the observed shunt of OLV in clinical studies is 20–28%.

Ventilation

The use of OLV and the adoption of the lateral decubitus position results in specific physiological changes, such as the shifts in West Zones from vertical to horizontal, which are best countered by positive pressure ventilation (see Table 7.4). It is physical forces mainly that must be dealt with – all these effectively summating to compress the FRC. The open pneumothorax, weight of mediastinum, abdominal contents on adoption of the lateral decubitus position and the surgeon at work compress the dependent lung; and, all must be opposed through the narrow conduit of, often, the single lumen of a DLT.

Simplistic though it may appear, it needs to be reiterated that the minute volume for OLV is that of normal two-lung ventilation. In compensating for the dynamics of OLV, some advocate for the routine a tidal volume of 8–10 ml/kg with appropri-

Table 7.4 The lung that does not collapse.

Stop ventilation
Aspirate with suction tracheal and bronchial lumen
Allow the lung to deflate with gentle decompression
Put more air into bronchial cuff (simple leak)
Reventilate with reduced driving pressure
If still a problem
Reposition endobronchial tube (use flexible bronchoscope)
Insert a blocker into the tracheal lumen of DLT and inflate (a Foley catheter has been used in the past)
or
Accept the situation and alternate surgery with ventilation

ate respiration frequency to maintain normocapnia. Increasingly, there has been recognition that the operative ventilation conditions are incriminated in post-operative pulmonary dysfunction. Others now recommend a peak inflation pressure limitation ($< 35 \, cm \, H_2O$) and the use of smaller tidal volumes (4–6 ml/kg). However, airway pressure parameters need to account for the increase in resistance of the small size DLT, and driving pressure increased appropriately. In extreme cases such as lung volume reduction and lung transplantation normocapnia may have to be sacrificed, and a degree of permissive hypercapnia accepted ($< 12 \, kPa$).

Common problems
Oxygen desaturation ($< 90\%$)

If hypoxia occurs once OLV has been satisfactorily established, the problems in Table 7.5 are sufficiently common in ranking or importance to be routinely checked for. Reference is to be made to Table 7.1 (first aid) while the cause of hypoxia is established and treated.

If these simple measures fail to correct hypoxia, consider recruiting the operative lung. The most common method is to employ a cPAP system, of which several are described, to the operative

Table 7.5 Physiological changes due to OLV.
Effects on hypoxic pulmonary vasoconstriction
Lung volume alterations
Atelectasis
Gas trapping in distal airways
Increased muscle activity
Decreased outward chest wall recoil
Increased elastic recoil of lung
Increased thoracic blood volume
Changes in airways resistance
Depression of ventilatory control mechanism

Table 7.6 Desaturation scenarios.
Separator moved. Tube "too far"; lobar bronchus blocked
Secretions in the endotracheal tube or DLT
Ventilated lung – FRC fall. Change driving pressure to compensate for small tracheal lumen
Muscle relaxant worn off (usually a late phenomenon)
Fall in cardiac output
Dynamic hyperinflation (disconnect ventilator)
Ipsilateral pneumothorax
Surgical cause (pressure on bronchus, mediastinum, PA or heart)

lung. Although this is usually done as a reaction to hypoxia, there is argument for using it proactively to reduce the risks of post-operative acute lung injury (ALI) through achieving gas exchange by overworking and over-stressing the ventilated lung.

Other methods have been suggested to reduce the shunt, such as soft clamping pulmonary artery or insertion and inflation of pulmonary artery balloon catheters. In general these are not recommended; there is significant risk of long-lasting damage. The concept of producing a chemical pneumonectomy circulation using vasoactive drugs has been suggested. The current drugs (nitric oxide, almatrine) are toxic and indiscriminate and the idea has little to recommend it for routine use.

Lung that does not collapse
Some of these events are, in practice, pathological rather than clinical with the presence of pleural adhesions a common culprit for this source of irritation to our surgical colleagues. Nevertheless, the ritual of trying to improve surgical conditions by manipulating the OLV system has to be undertaken (see Table 7.4).

Re-inflation problems
Usually, the lung re-inflates once the tracheal lumen is ventilated. The most common reason for difficulty re-inflating a lung is the herniated bronchial cuff obstructing the contralateral bronchus. A graduated response is required. Ultimately it may be necessary to deflate the bronchial cuff and apply extra manual driving pressure. This may be an occasion that warrants the use of a fiberoptic bronchoscope to confirm or discount this problem.

Special considerations
Positive end-expiratory pressure (PEEP)
The reduction in FRC and closing volume that is further exacerbated by the effects of decubitus position potentially can lead to atelectasis and is influenced by PEEP. The clinical evidence is that it is not necessary as routine and indeed may be harmful: the effects on right ventricular function and cardiac output potentially exaggerated. In the event of oxygen desaturation those with clear evidence of background obstructive airways disease should be considered. However, it is a trial and error exercise.

The use of high frequency ventilation techniques has been attempted. There may be occasional circumstances such as the presence of broncho-pleural fistulae, or in emphysema, but studies have shown no benefit to justify a routine use of complex equipment. There remains the enhanced risk for a vibrating PEEP dynamic being generated with volu-trauma and barotrauma of friable pulmonary tissue and circulation.

Dynamic hyperinflation

One of the main consequences of operating on patients for lung transplantation and lung vol-ume reduction with background of emphysema-tous lung disease is the frequent occurrence of dynamic hyperinflation due to air trapping on insti-tution of positive pressure ventilation. It is impor-tant to recognize the precursors of this rapidly fatal complication, which are the combination of an acute fall in oxygenation and blood pressure. The test effect of disconnecting the ventilator and rapid resolution is pathognomic. A protective form of ventilation should be instituted with peak inflation reduced to < 20 cm H_2O fall and a prolonged expi-ratory time of I:E ratio 1:>3. Permissive hypercap-nia may be necessary and frequent periods of apnea with ventilator disconnection required to tide over the crisis.

Terminating OLV

It is axiomatic in this field that the ventilation sys-tem most appropriate and safe for a patient is spon-taneous respiration. This is an early and prime goal. In these authors' practice, tracheal extubation is conducted with the patient still anesthetized and preceded by careful suction to ensure secretions and debris at the carina are not inhaled.

FURTHER READING

- Brunelli A, Pieretti P, Refai M *et al.* Elective intensive care after lung resection: a multicentric propensity-matched comparison of outcome. *Interact CardioVasc Thorac Surg* 2005; **4**: 609–13.
- Cohen E. Anesthetic management of one-lung ventilation. *Pract Thorac Anesth* 1995; 308–40.
- Conacher ID. Dynamic hyperinflation – the anaesthetist applying a tourniquet to the right heart. *Br J Anaesth* 1998; **81**: 116–17.
- Conacher ID. Time to apply Occam's razor to HPV during one-lung ventilation. *Br J Anaesth* 2000; **84**: 434–5.
- Conacher ID. Postoperative pulmonary oedema-tussles with starlings in the death zone. *Anaesthesia* 2006; **61(3)**: 211–14.
- Cook DJ. Practical management of one-lung anesthesia. *Revista Mexicana de Anestesiologica* 2005; **28(S1)**: S54–64.
- Kaplan JA, Slinger PD. *Thoracic Anesthesia*, 3rd edn. 2003.
- Pfitzner J. A new clinical sign during one-lung-anaesthesia: fact or fiction? *Anaesthesia* 2002; **57(3)**: 293–4.
- Slinger PD. Postpneumonectomy pulmonary edema: good news, bad news. *Anesthesiology* 2006; **105**: 2–5.
- Slinger PD. Pro: low tidal volume is indicated during one-lung ventilation. *Anesth Analg* 2006; **103(2)**: 268–70.

Section 2 Anesthesia for operative procedures

Chapter 8

Anesthetic implications of bronchoscopy

IAN CONACHER

Rigid bronchoscopic removal of inhaled foreign bodies has been a constant theme for a century. It will continue to be so. Rigid bronchoscopy (RB) was a necessary art of assessment of fitness for lung resection surgery and placing lung separator devices (LSD) (large foreign bodies!). Effective use of endobronchial blockers (e.g. Vernon–Thompson) and endobronchial tubes (e.g. Macintosh–Leatherdale, Brompton–Pallister) depended on expertise particularly for left lung isolation. The requirement was lessened as surgery shifted from that of tuberculosis to that of cancer and the role of the anesthetist shifted to peri-operative and post-operative conduct. But there remains a core of conditions where the essence of operational and therapeutic process is anesthesia for RB. And, RB technology has been – and continues to be – modified, for interventions such as lasers and tracheo-bronchial stents (Figure 8.1).

For the practice of the modern thoracic anesthetist, the differences between RB and fiberoptic bronchoscopic (FOB) instrumentation are brought in to focus by the new technologies. Principally, these relate to RB as conduits for tools versus FOB in diagnostics. The latter are the dominant device for insertion of bronchial blockers (e.g. Univent, Arndt, Cohen) and elucidating lung separator problems. Rigid bronchoscopy, by enabling gas exchange at the same time as the variety of instrument changes and maneuvers, has a new lease and gives a constancy that has facilitated the therapeutic advances for the endoscopic management of tracheal and endobronchial pathology. Those whose professional lives will be dominated by fiberoptic technology should be aware of the illusions that can be created by taking shortcuts with lessons learnt from the art of RB. Time spent observing latter day masters and acquiring a working skill will not be amiss for the 21st-century thoracic anesthetist. The particular value is in the importance of gaining knowledge of the true value of the "sniffing the morning air" position for sight and access to the larynx.

Anesthesia for bronchoscopy

Rigid bronchoscope insertion is very stimulating. A large, even massive pressor response is generated. Anesthesia must take account of this in a patient's fitness for process assessment and, if not ablate it, at least obtund it. The risks of hemodynamic, cardiac or cerebral complications are significant particularly in a case-mix likely to be preconditioned with allied comorbidities.

Non-anesthetists practise most FOB. Local anethesia is applied topically when advancing the scope. Increasingly, in context, FOB are passed

Core Topics in Thoracic Anesthesia, ed. Cait P. Searl and Sameena T. Ahmed. Published by Cambridge University Press.
© Cambridge University Press 2009.

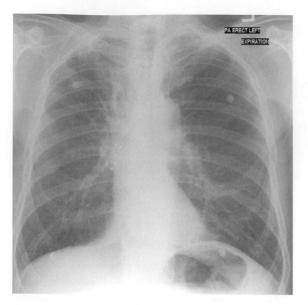

Figure 8.1 A chest X-ray showing a stent in position in the right main bronchus.

through RB under general anesthesia. Nevertheless, local and regional techniques for RB should not be discounted, particularly for the very sick in whom preserving of consciousness and self-ventilation is paramount. Organe, writing 60 years ago, describes the experience of RB under local anesthesia. So artfully can this be done that this eminent anesthetist was able to state: it was preferable to "going to the dentist."

For RB, general anesthesia is the norm. For short procedures a propofol and opioid supplemented (alfentanil, fentanyl) induction is a usual regimen, followed by a short-acting non-depolarizing agent such as mivacurium. There remains an occasional need (e.g. managing broncho-pleural fistulae) for suxamethonium. This should be preceded by pre-curarization to prevent fasciculations causing fouling of a lung that is vulnerable until a secure ventilation system is in place.

Rigid endoscopy, in general, had a bad record of awareness. By any measure this is no longer acceptable but it is less likely. Propofol is protective but until confidence in such advances as bispectral index (BIS) and entropy monitors are established, it is wise to include benzodiazepine prophylaxis e.g. midazolam, either as premedication or on induction for the diagnostic or short process.

For more prolonged procedures, total intravenous anesthesia (TIVA) has proved remarkable. Propofol and remifentanil by controlled infusion are the local standard. Pressor response ablation and hemodynamic stability are easily achieved for the periods of stimulation that result from protracted processes that are in the nature of foreign body removal, tracheal and bronchial laser resection and tracheo-bronchial stenting, despite often intense competition for the airway from therapists and anesthetist. Mivacurium as an adjunct for muscle relaxation is proving satisfactory and has the merit of not often requiring the use of reversal agents. There are mixed messages about the use of topical anesthesia as supplement. The author's view is that its use does not add any benefit and in the unfit may interfere with recovery (*vide infra*).

Positive pressure ventilation

Manufacturers of current equipment pay little attention to the needs of patient ventilation during operation of their devices. The concessions are small and at the operational end, employing one of three attachments which make positive pressure ventilation possible, but only just!

1. A Luer fitting for jet or Sanders' type.
2. A port for attachment of a jet or high frequency jet ventilator.
3. An attachment for an anesthetic system in conjunction with a cap that fits on the top of the bronchoscope to seal the system so that volatile agents also can be used in addition to continuous-flow oxygen or air. A clear window and fenestrated slide (to allow instrument insertion) sometimes are integral to the cap attachment. This set up is referred to as a ventilating bronchoscope.

Jet systems can be relatively uncontrolled; not uncommonly close to direct pipeline pressure. Overinflation of lungs, barotrauma and air trapping are potential dangers to be alert to. End-tidal CO_2 monitoring is difficult and all things withstanding generally is dispensed with.

In an emergency the suction port can be used for jet ventilation. If all else fails, a standard tracheal tube can be jammed into the top of an RB and the patient oxygenated from a reservoir bag by hand.

Emerging from the anesthetic

The termination of a procedure can be difficult: recovery of cough reflex and consciousness protracted and complicated. Sick patients are destabilized by the excess of pharmacology and surgical manipulation so that delicate and precarious physiological adaptations to their airway pathology may be slow to re-establish. Carbon dioxide retention may follow. The recovery end point is the cough. *"The cough and nothing but the cough"* in its entirety must be heard and seen to have been retrieved before the patient is safe – *"so help me cough"* is a good mantra in this endeavor! Coordinated deep inspiration, the closed glottis and forced expectorating expiration are the gold standard of criteria for transfer to recovery. Secretions, blood clot, tumor, laser debris and pus lurk in the depths ready to obstruct without warning. Reinsertion of an RB commonly (10%) is an urgent requirement; and a recovery period of IPPV an occasional one.

Rigid bronchoscopy for major events
Airway obstruction

Intrinsic and extrinsic lesions of the trachea can present as life-threatening emergencies. Some patients are in such dire straits that the energy to generate telltale stridor is not possible. First aid measures include airway humidification, steroids on an empirical basis, and inspiration of helium oxygen mixes until an RB can be inserted. There is an experience-base that a rapid sequence inser-tion of the RB is least likely, in contrast to gas induction sequences, to precipitate total obstruction. Oxygen can be forced past the obstruction: in so doing it must be remembered that the risk of creating dynamic hyperinflation is significant. Nevertheless, the presence of an RB then allows for accurate assessment of the situation, the potential of a variety of treatment options and physical interventions, all within a relatively efficient gas-exchanging environment. The work up to tracheal resection and decisions for management of the airway during transection are best made on bronchoscopic findings.

Difficult intubation

Before the fiberoptic revolution, difficult airways were not so common but nevertheless occurred. Early photographs by pioneers of RB clearly illustrate that the "sniffing the morning air" position was naturally adopted by those whose operating tables were little more than wooden platforms with an assistant to support the occiput of the patient in the optimum position to avoid esophageal intubation. The straight blade laryngoscope design unconsciously followed on this experience. Thus one of the stratagems to deal with the difficult airway was to use an RB; for even if the trachea is not cannulated there is an easy route to place a bougie over which to railroad a tracheal tube. Oxygenation can be prevented from developing to hazardous levels by intermittent jet ventilation directed along the RB.

Hemoptysis

The erosion of a major vessel in the bronchial tree occasionally results in unstoppable hemoptysis. With much of the cardiac output coming up an RB, it is impossible to do anything to intervene. However, most bleeds are small and temporary but surprisingly difficult to define. Rigid bronchoscopy is necessary at some point in diagnosis or therapy. Acute hemorrhage (e.g. post biopsy) is best dealt with by tamponade with an adrenaline-soaked pledget on an applicator through the RB, while gas exchange is assisted by a jet or Sanders' type device and directed to the non-afflicted lung. Airway and visibility in the area are maintained, enough for holding measures, such as double lumen tubes or bronchial blockers, to be applied.

Broncho-pleural fistula

Most are pin-hole leaks presenting post-operatively, through which the contents of a pneumonectomy-space leak to cause infection and aspiration in the remnant lung. The totally blown bronchial stump case, rare though it is, is a stereotype for an RB method of management. In this model, up to a liter of pus may be present in the space. The first aid measure is to attempt to drain, via an intercostal space, as much of the pneumonectomy space as possible but to be aware that this may not be sufficient to prevent loculated fluid entering the trachea.

1. Sit the patient up and tilt them to the side of the lesion.
2. Pre-oxygenate, precurarize (to prevent fasciculations), induce (etomidate) and then administer suxamethonium.
3. With the onset of apnea introduce the RB. Under direct vision observe the fistula, aspirate any contaminants with a large-bore suction attachment, place the tip of the bronchoscope in the non-affected bronchus and ventilate.
4. If lung isolation is required, pass an airway exchange catheter into the non-affected bronchus, remove the RB and "rail-road" an endobronchial or double-lumen tube into position.

Foreign bodies

Almost anything, small enough, can be inhaled. Toy whistles, bits of Christmas tree, Biro caps, chicken gristle are amongst the exotica seen by the author in addition to a diet of peanuts, pins and dentistry. A variety of instruments or contraptions may have to be employed. Extraction can be prolonged, and

fiddly but all are made feasible by an anesthetic technique centered on the rigid scope and TIVA.

Rigid bronchoscopy for the emergent technologies

Cryoprobes, lasers, and tracheo-bronchial stents have in succession evolved from the cumbersome to the convenient. The case-mix contains the most challenging of patients, frequently with major airway pathology, in respiratory failure, with a background of symptomatic comorbidities of cardio-respiratory disease. These situations are best done using both RB (to secure airway and ventilate) and FOB (to treat and apply therapy options). Although FOB access means that primary care with laser or stents can be done without access to RB, the latter indisputably remains necessary when problems arise.

First aid measures include positioning of the patient, humidification, non-invasive positive pressure ventilation and inhalation use of helium oxygen mix. Most will have been given steroids empirically. The use of local anesthesia supplementation is tempting. However, this does delay the re-establishment of the full and efficient cough reflex.

Lasers in the airway

The real attribute of the RB in the situation of operating lasers in the airway is the metal construction. This reduces the fire hazard, a risk never totally negated. The modern fiber delivery laser instruments are small enough to be inserted through a FOB, enabling a combined rigid/fiberoptic system that extends laser treatment options further into the airway and for more complex lesions. However, the plastic material of FOB is a hazard: it is ignitable by the laser fiber. It is thus mandatory that the RB is ventilated by an **air** (21% oxygen) driven system so that a sequence that potentially leads to fire or explosion is not initiated.

Box 8.1 Learning points

1. In thoracic anesthetic practice rigid and fiberoptic bronchoscopy are complementary, not alternatives.
2. There is significant pressor response to the presence of a bronchoscope.
3. There is a risk of awareness.
4. Jet ventilation systems are efficient but there are options.
5. Problems in thoracic practice are more easily solved when viewed as situations of anesthesia and ventilation for rigid bronchoscopy.
6. Fire in the airway is always a risk when lasers are used.
7. Fiberoptic bronchoscopes can delude and create inappropriate mindsets.
8. Once the airway is secure, make an opportunity to experience esophageal intubation with a flexible fiberoptic bronchoscope.

Stents

The advent of self-expanding devices has considerably eased the burden of sharing access to the airway with surgeons or physicians. The latter can make adjustments with FOB or rigid end viewing fiberscopes. A few patients still require Montgomery or solid wall stents, with RB of necessity both for insertion and maintenance of life during the procedure and periodic servicing.

Words about fiberoptics (Box 8.1)
LIMITATIONS

The optics of the FOB are unrivalled enabling sight of subsegmental bronchi: the RB limited by bulk and poorer optics to major bronchi. However, diagnostically there are some features which are not emulated by FOB.

1. Depth of field. With FOB this is difficult. Illustrated by the need to get some sense surgically of clear margins at the point of bronchotomy – sometimes the difference between a lobectomy or a pneumonectomy.

2. The inoperable tumor, bronchogenic or esophageal, causes a characteristic rigidity that can be sensed with an RB.

AS A TOOL

An earlier generation commonly were faced with being unable to correct a misplaced tube or use an endobronchial tube without having to disengage it from a main bronchus: conditions of lung separation were difficult to re-establish. The FOB to diagnose and site problems and to be used as a railroad guide is a great boon and valuable aid.

WORDS OF WARNING

The illusion of a correctly sited lung separator such as a double lumen tube is easily created. A CEPOD assessment found that the left-sided tube incorrectly sited and not being detected as in the right main bronchus was probably contributory to several operative deaths. It was apparent that this misplacement could inspire a sense of correct siting which would be confirmed by FOB. A correct process of anticipation (10% of left-sided tubes will tend to enter the right main bronchus), observation and auscultation in sequence before use of the FOB helps ensure that this illusion does not get created in the minds of the anesthetist.

FURTHER READING

- Conacher ID. Anaesthesia and tracheobronchial stenting for central airway obstruction in adults. *Br J Anaesth* 2003; **90(3)**: 367–74.
- Conacher ID, Curran E. Local anaesthesia and sedation for rigid bronchoscopy for emergency relief of central airway obstruction. *Anaesthesia* 2004; **59**: 290–2.
- Håkanson E, Konstantinov IE, Fransson S-G, Svedjeholm R. Management of life threatening haemoptysis. *Br J Anaesth* 2002; **88(2)**: 291–5.
- Organe G. Personal experience of bronchoscopy. *Proc Roy Soc Med* 1946; **39**: 635–6.

Chapter 9

Anesthesia for tracheal surgery

TAJ DHALLU

Historically, surgery on the trachea in the form of tracheostomy has been carried out for at least 2000 years. However, it was not until the 1960s that tracheal surgery was developed and advanced in order to manage the increasing number of patients with tracheal stenosis. There was little experience of operating on tumors of the trachea whether malignant or benign because of their rarity.

The development of modern anesthesia techniques involving the ventilation of the patient's lungs and the use of tracheal tubes in intensive care and anesthesia was a great impetus to the development of surgery in general. The use of these early tracheal tubes resulted in some cases to damage of the trachea and its subsequent stenosis; once the complications of endotracheal tubes were appreciated there was not only a rapid development of tracheal surgery but also of the design of tracheal tubes. The other factor that limited the development of tracheal surgery was the belief by surgeons that only two to three tracheal rings could be excised.

Although tracheal surgery is only carried out in specialized centers, all anesthetists will benefit from the understanding of the principles of management of this difficult airway and what is possible in modern anesthesia. The most important requirement for surgery on the trachea is that the surgeon and anesthetist need to be able to communicate with each other as there is a high risk of not being able to oxygenate the patient and disaster occurring. This communication should start well before the patient arrives in theater and both surgeon and anesthetist need to understand what the other will be doing at every stage of the procedure.

The types of procedures carried out on the trachea that require general anesthesia are rigid bronchoscopy, tracheal stenting and excision of tracheal stenosis or tumors.

Rigid bronchoscopy

Rigid bronchoscopy can be used for diagnostic purposes by examining and assessing the tracheobronchial tree anatomy and by the taking of a biopsy for histology. The clearing of mucus plugs or clots, the excision or laser ablation of intratracheobronchial masses and the placement of stents are important roles of the rigid bronchoscope. The conduct of anesthesia for this has been discussed in the previous chapter.

Tracheal stenting

Tracheal stenosis, which cannot be corrected by surgery, may be amenable to stenting. Stents are devices to maintain patency of the lumen of the trachea or bronchi and can be placed for benign or malignant lesions. Stents can be made of

Core Topics in Thoracic Anesthesia, ed. Cait P. Searl and Sameena T. Ahmed. Published by Cambridge University Press.
© Cambridge University Press 2009.

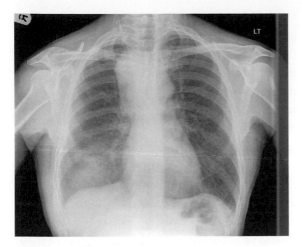

Figure 9.1 A chest X-ray showing tracheal stents in position.

silicone rubber or metal. Silicone rubber stents require general anesthesia for placement while metallic expandable stents can be placed fluoroscopically or under general anesthesia. Expandable stents are thin walled and do not interfere with ciliary function, but once placed are difficult to move. Expandable stents come collapsed on an introducer; when placed in the trachea or bronchi and released they expand and support the trachea (Figure 9.1). Under general anesthesia stents are placed with a rigid bronchoscope. The main complication is migration of the stent leading to the further obstruction of the airway. Malignant tumors may eventually occlude the stent.

Tracheal resection

The development and advance of tracheal surgery since the 1960s is due to Grillo and others. Up to 50% of the trachea can be resected and reconstructed. The indications for tracheal resection are symptomatic stenosis or benign and malignant tumors. Tracheal stenosis is most often caused by trauma such as prolonged intubation of the trachea in the intensive care unit; however, it is not always necessary that intubation be prolonged. Blunt trauma to the trachea can also cause the tra-

chea to be stenosed in an acute and chronic setting. There are also congenital causes of tracheal stenosis that may present in adult life.

Pathophysiology of tracheal stenosis

The tracheal stenosis may be fixed or dynamic. Fixed tracheal stenosis results in resistance to flow of air on inspiration and expiration. In dynamic tracheal stenosis there is weakening of the wall of the trachea at the stenosis so that the diameter of the stenosis depends upon the position of the stenosis, whether it is intrathoracic or extrathoracic and also upon inspiration or expiration.

If the tracheal stenosis is intrathoracic then upon inspiration the extratracheal pressure drops below that in the trachea, resulting in widening of the stenosis, and inspiration becomes easier, while upon expiration the increase in extratracheal pressure will be greater than that in the trachea and will tend to collapse the trachea, making expiration difficult.

If the tracheal stenosis is extrathoracic then upon inspiration the intratracheal pressure is below that of the extratracheal, thus the trachea narrows making inspiration difficult; upon expiration intratracheal pressure is higher than extratracheal, resulting in widening of the trachea and expiration becomes easier.

Management and preparation for tracheal resection

Once the tracheal stenosis is narrowed to less than 6 mm, the patient will experience increasing dyspnea, wheezing and stridor made worse by exercise. Forced expiratory volumes will become reduced and there will be a rise in the $PaCO_2$. Pre-operative investigations will attempt to obtain as much information as possible about the anatomy and extent of the obstruction. Flow volume loops will be flattened in expiration or inspiration or both depending upon the type of stenosis and its position.

With postero-anterior chest films along with a computerized axial tomography (CAT) scan, or spiral CT scanning of the thorax, a detailed three-dimensional picture can be built of the tracheo-bronchial tree and its relations.

Fiberoptic bronchoscopy under local anesthesia and possible biopsy if indicated will also allow one to visualize the extent and behavior of the stenosis and obtain tissue for histology.

If the tracheal stenosis is severe a rigid bronchoscopy under general anesthesia is appropriate, especially if there is a risk of complete airway obstruction; the rigid bronchoscope can be pushed past the obstruction to provide the airway. There may also be the possibility of dilating the stenosis with bougies or of debulking any tumors for palliation or before more extensive surgery. Historically, local anesthesia with nerve blocks has been carried out for rigid bronchoscopy, but it was not pleasant for the patient and difficult for the surgeon.

In preparing the patients for tracheal excision, apart from making them as medically fit as possible it is essential that patients are well motivated and understand that post-operatively they will need to maintain the head in flexion for up to a week in order not to put a strain on the tracheal sutures and to allow healing.

When embarking upon anesthesia it is vital that the surgeon and anesthetist discuss all the steps of surgery and anesthesia especially where there may be a risk of loss of control of the airway. Plans should be ready for all eventualities. Sterile armored tracheal tubes, Montandon tubes, ventilator tubing along with equipment for jet ventilation should all be immediately to hand. Jet ventilator can be a Sanders injector or one of the more sophisticated jet ventilators that are available.

The surgical incision will depend upon the position of the stenosis or tumor. Incisions used are thoracotomy, median sternotomy, cervical collar or a combination of these. It is important to realize that these incisions can be extended many ways.

The requirements of general anesthesia are that there should be a smooth induction with a technique that allows the trachea to be extubated in theatre post-operatively. Thus the use of minimal opioids along with a volatile agent such as sevoflurane would be suitable.

The patient would have had rigid bronchoscopy in the pre-assessment period and one would proceed with this knowledge in mind. An intra-arterial cannula in a radial artery should be placed for beat-to-beat blood pressure measurement and to monitor arterial blood gases while a pulse oximeter probe should be placed on the other hand. Either of these monitors will register an alteration of pulse wave should the innominate artery be inadvertently compressed by the surgeon. Thoracic epidural should be considered for a thoracotomy incision.

We routinely insert a naso-gastric tube after general anesthesia in most of our thoracic patients in order to decompress the stomach in order to prevent regurgitation and splinting of the diaphragm by air post-operatively.

Intubation of the trachea with an armored tube will secure the airway. If the stenosis is minor then the tracheal tube can be passed beyond, but surgery is made more difficult because the tracheal tube gets in the way of surgery, especially when the surgeon needs to put sutures at the posterior aspect of the trachea.

Once the surgeon has carried out the initial median sternotomy or thoracotomy then further dissection will be carried out to release the trachea from the surrounding tissues in order to provide length to the trachea and reduce tension on tracheal anastomotic sutures. Once the trachea is released the surgeon will want to transect the trachea below the stenosis or tumor, at this point it is vital that the patient has been pre-oxygenated with 100% oxygen and that the scrub staff have a range of armored tracheal tubes along with sterile ventilator tubing. When the surgeon is ready to transect the trachea, the oral tracheal tube is withdrawn to just below the vocal cords, the surgeon will transect the trachea and place a sterile tracheal tube of a suitable diameter in the distal trachea; this is connected to sterile ventilator tubing which is handed to the anesthetist who will connect it to the ventilator and ventilate the patient's lungs.

Once the stenosis or tumor is excised the surgeon will start to anastamose the trachea. At this point the head of the patient will need to be flexed and maintained – this can be achieved with the use of pillows. On nearing completion of the anastamosis the distal tracheal tube will need to be removed by the surgeon and ventilation of the lungs re-commenced through the oral tracheal tube. At this moment the anesthetist must be ready to again ventilate through the distal tracheal tube if it needs to be reinserted because of problems with the anastamosis.

After completion of the anastamosis it can be assessed from the inside of the trachea with a fiberoptic scope and the chest closed. Finally the surgeon will place sutures from the patient's chin to the chest to maintain neck flexion. The chin-to-chest sutures are removed after 7 days.

It cannot be emphasized too much to say that it is essential that the patient is only extubated when fully awake and able to maintain the airway and it is absolutely essential to maintain flexion of the neck with pressure at the back of the head if necessary. This can be a difficult time in a semi-conscious patient. Upon extubation of the trachea the vocal cords are examined with a fiberoptic scope as the

tracheal tube and the scope are withdrawn in order to determine if there has been recurrent laryngeal nerve injury. Re-intubation will be difficult with the neck in flexion, thus we leave a catheter in the trachea after extubation just in case we need to railroad the tracheal tube back into the trachea. We remain in theater with the patient until we are confident that the patient is awake and cooperative and can then be transferred to the intensive care unit. Humidified oxygen is administered.

Carinal resection would follow the above principles, but is more complicated as one may require the placement of either tracheal tubes or jet ventilation catheters in both bronchi.

Conclusion

Surgery on the trachea requires that the surgeon and anesthetist have excellent communication and rapport in order to avoid loss of control of the airway. Thorough understanding of the nature and anatomy of the tracheal lesion is essential for safe anesthesia.

FURTHER READING

- Grillo HC. *Surgery of the Trachea and Bronchi.* Decker BC, 2003.
- Magnusson L, Lang FJ, Monnier P, *et al.* Anaesthesia for tracheal resection. *Can J Anaesth* 1997; 44: 1282–5.
- Pinsonneault C, Fortier J, Donati F, *et al.* Tracheal resection and reconstruction. *Can J Anesth* 1997; 46: 439–55.

Chapter 10

Anesthesia for mediastinoscopy and mediastinal surgery

DAVID C. SMITH

The prognosis for patients with mediastinal pathology has improved significantly in recent years as a result of better understanding of the impact of chemotherapy and radiotherapy on malignant mediastinal tumors. However, diagnostic biopsy and subsequent tumor resection are still hazardous procedures. In contrast, although thymectomy is still a major undertaking in patients with myasthenia gravis, fewer patients now require prolonged post-operative respiratory support as a result of improved understanding of the disease.

Mediastinal anatomy

The mediastinum is the space in the center of the chest bounded by the plurae on either side, the sternum anteriorly and the thoracic vertebral column posteriorly (Figure 10.1). The upper boundary is the thoracic inlet, and the lower boundary is the diaphragm. It is divided into superior and inferior portions by a line joining the sternal angle to the fourth thoracic vertebra. The inferior portion is further divided into anterior, middle and posterior parts (Table 10.1).

Mediastinal pathology

The relative incidence of mediastinal masses is given in Table 10.2. Approximately 90% of lymph node masses in the mediastinum are metastatic.

The signs and symptoms of mediastinal pathology range from trivial to life-threatening, and include airway compression, superior vena cava syndrome, compression of the right heart and pulmonary arteries, and dysphagia from esophageal compression (Table 10.3). Venous obstruction is a particular problem, because the smaller veins expand to allow collateral flow, increasing the risk of bleeding during anesthetic or surgical instrumentation. Neural compression is also common, and may produce severe pain, vocal cord palsy (recurrent laryngeal nerve) or Horner's syndrome.

In order to establish a firm diagnosis in mediastinal disease it is important to obtain a tissue biopsy, because many of these lesions are malignant and the decision to use radiotherapy, chemotherapy or a combination of these, is highly tumor-dependent.

Assessment of patients for mediastinal surgery

Many mediastinal masses are asymptomatic, and are discovered during routine examination or chest radiography. Most lesions in asymptomatic patients are benign, whilst symptomatic lesions are frequently malignant, although large masses tend to produce more severe symptoms irrespective of the pathology. Patients may therefore present for mediastinal surgery in a range of conditions, but the

Core Topics in Thoracic Anesthesia, ed. Cait P. Searl and Sameena T. Ahmed. Published by Cambridge University Press.
© Cambridge University Press 2009.

Table 10.1 Contents of the mediastinum.

Superior	Inferior
Aortic arch and branches	*Anterior*
Innominate vein	Lymph nodes
Superior vena cava	*Middle*
Trachea	Heart
Esophagus	Ascending aorta
Thoracic duct	Pulmonary vessels
Thymus	Superior vena cava
Recurrent laryngeal nerves	Phrenic and vagus nerves
Lymph nodes	Lymph nodes
	Posterior
Retrosternal extension of the thyroid	Main bronchi
	Esophagus
	Descending aorta
	Azygos veins
	Thoracic duct
	Lymph nodes

Table 10.2 Incidence of mediastinal mass lesions.

Neurogenic tumor	20%	Usually posterior
Thymoma	19%	30% have myasthenia
Cysts	18%	Pericardial 6%, Bronchogenic 6%
Lymphoma	13%	Usually anterior or middle mediastinum
Germ cell tumor	10%	
Mesenchymal tumor	6%	
Endocrine tumor	6%	
Primary carcinoma	5%	

Table 10.3 Symptoms in mediastinal disease.

Chest pain	30–40%
Dyspnea	22%
Cough	18–40%
Fever	13–24%
Weight loss	9–24%
SVC syndrome	8–16%
Myasthenia gravis	7%
Fatigue	6%
Dysphagia	4%
Night sweats	3%

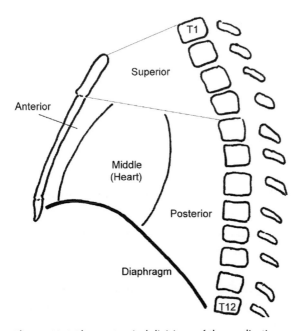

Figure 10.1 The anatomical divisions of the mediastinum.

principal problems for the anesthetist are difficulties with airway management, potentially complex surgery if tumors are being resected and the risk of major hemorrhage. Significant weight loss is unusual, and these patients are no more prone to endocrine or cardiovascular abnormalities than other patients. The surgical approach for diagnostic procedures is via cervical mediastinoscopy or anterior mediastinotomy, while for tumor resection the usual approaches are via median sternotomy or lateral thoracotomy.

Inhalation

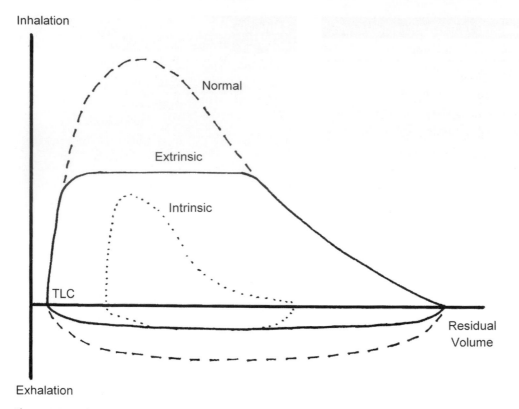

Exhalation

Figure 10.2 Spirometry in airways obstruction. The effort-dependent part of the expiratory curve reaches a plateau in the case of extrinsic airways compression, whilst it has a concave appearance in intrinsic airways obstruction such as chronic obstructive pulmonary disease. Erect and supine spirometry enables identification of those patients in whom extrinsic compression of the airways only occurs on lying down. TLC, total lung capacity.

Careful evaluation of the airway is necessary during pre-operative assessment for surgery within the mediastinum. Chest X-ray, including thoracic inlet views when necessary, and thoracic computerized tomographs should be studied for evidence of airway compression or displacement. Occasionally it may be difficult to decide whether respiratory symptoms result from intrinsic or extrinsic airway disease. In these patients erect and supine spirometry may be helpful (Figure 10.2). Although radiotherapy and chemotherapy have improved the prognosis of mediastinal tumors and enabled tumor mass to be reduced before definitive surgery, these treatments often obscure the tissue diagnosis, which is crucial to further management of the disease. It is possible to shield a portion of the tumor from the radiation beam, reducing symptoms while leaving a portion of the tumor unaffected by radiation, but this approach is uncommon and these patients often present for mediastinoscopy with significant respiratory or vascular obstruction.

The patient presenting for mediastinal surgery may also have systemic disease as a result of chemotherapy. Doxorubicin may produce a dose-related cardiomyopathy, especially if the dose exceeds 500 mg/m^2. Bleomycin may give rise to post-operative respiratory failure in association with high inspired oxygen concentrations, especially in patients over 70 years of age or who have received more than 400 units of bleomycin.

Myelodysplasia is a side-effect of most chemotherapeutic agents.

Anesthesia for cervical mediastinoscopy

Mediastinoscopy is usually performed to obtain a tissue diagnosis for mediastinal tumors, and to stage, or determine the operability of, other intrathoracic tumors. It was first described by Carlens in 1959, and provides information which would otherwise require thoracotomy.

The patient's head is placed on a head ring and the neck is fully extended. The upper half of the patient is tilted slightly head-up to reduce venous engorgement, although this maneuver slightly increases the risk of air embolism during the procedure. Access for the mediastinoscope is through a small incision above the suprasternal notch, followed by blunt dissection through the pretracheal fascia and behind the manubrium into the superior mediastinum between the trachea and the aortic arch.

Mediastinoscopy is a short procedure which is often performed immediately following a diagnostic bronchoscopy. It may be performed under local anesthesia, but general anesthesia is more commonly used. Although it is feasible to allow the patient to breathe spontaneously during mediastinoscopy, even via a laryngeal mask, tracheal intubation and positive pressure ventilation is a safer approach which also minimizes the risk of air embolism through open mediastinal veins. Endobronchial intubation is not indicated for mediastinoscopy, although an armored tracheal tube may be useful to prevent kinking of the tube during the procedure.

The choice of induction technique may be dictated by pre-existing respiratory compromise, and inhalation induction may be the safest approach in selected patients. The maintenance anesthetic agents and neuromuscular blocking drugs should be chosen to enable a rapid return to consciousness, so that the patient may be safely extubated at the end of the procedure.

A large-bore intravenous cannula should be inserted, because of the risk of major hemorrhage, and if there is superior vena caval obstruction the cannula should be sited in a leg vein. Recommended minimal monitoring standards should be observed. The blood pressure cuff or arterial cannula, as appropriate, may best be sited on the left arm since compression of the right-sided head and neck vessels is common during mediastinoscopy. However, placement of an arterial cannula or pulse oximeter on the right arm may help to identify arterial compression, though this approach will often provide misleading pressure readings; palpation of the right radial artery during the procedure is an alternative approach.

Complications of mediastinoscopy

Death as a result of mediastinoscopy is unusual (around 0.1%), but the complication rate is 1.5–3% and complications may require rapid intervention (Table 10.4). The commonest complication is bleeding, and blood should be readily available. Although catastrophic bleeding is rare, its control may require emergency sternotomy or lateral thoracotomy. Effective fluid resuscitation may require vascular access in a leg vein if a large mediastinal

Table 10.4 Complications of mediastinoscopy.	
Common	**Unusual**
Hemorrhage	Infection
Pneumothorax	Tumor implantation
Recurrent laryngeal nerve injury	Phrenic nerve injury
Arterial compression	Esophageal injury
Tracheal compression	Air embolism
Dysrhythmia	Chylothorax
	Stroke

vein is damaged. Pneumothorax is also common, but does not often require a chest drain. Damage to the recurrent laryngeal nerve may occur, especially on the left side, and this may be permanent in 50% of cases. It is impractical to assess vocal cord function routinely at the end of the procedure, but a high index of suspicion is required as bilateral recurrent nerve injury may result in airway obstruction. Arterial compression is also common, and may cause cerebral hypoperfusion and transient or permanent cerebral damage, especially in patients with cerebrovascular disease. Compression of the aortic arch may cause a reflex bradycardia.

Anesthesia for anterior mediastinotomy

Anterior mediastinotomy is performed via a small incision to the left of the sternum, through the second intercostal space or the bed of the second costal cartilage. This approach permits examination of anterior mediastinal structures, especially the thymus, which are inaccessible during cervical mediastinoscopy. It is also a convenient route for open lung biopsy. Although anterior mediastinotomy is an extrapleural procedure, pleural tears are common and a small pneumothorax is common. A post-operative chest X-ray is therefore advisable, but a chest drain is not often required. Anesthetic considerations are the same as for cervical mediastinoscopy.

Anesthesia for resection of mediastinal masses

Access to mediastinal structures may be via median sternotomy (sometimes limited hemisternotomy) or lateral thoracotomy. Anesthetic considerations are the same as those for mediastinoscopy, as mentioned above, except that a double-lumen endobronchial tube will be required for lateral thoracotomy. Surgery will often be complex and bloody. Steps should be taken to maintain normothermia,

and consideration should be given to forced air warming blankets and warming systems for intravenous fluids.

Myasthenia gravis

Myasthenia gravis is an autoimmune disease in which IgG auto-antibodies destroy the postsynaptic nicotinic acetylcholine receptors of the motor endplate, reducing the number of functional receptors by about 70–80%. The reduced number of receptors eliminates the margin of safety in neuromuscular transmission and results in rapid muscle fatigue, the clinical presentation depending on the muscle groups affected (Table 10.5). Antibodies to acetylcholine receptors are present in 90% of patients with myasthenia, but it is the antibody activity, rather than the titer in plasma, which predicts the severity of the disease. Diagnostically the muscle fatigue is reversed by a small dose of edrophonium (the Tensilon test). The incidence of myasthenia in the population is around 1:30 000, with a 3:2 female:male preponderance; the peak incidence in women is in the third decade, while in men it is in the fifth decade.

Myasthenia is commonly associated with other autoimmune disorders. A thymoma is common (around 50%) but patients without thymoma will usually have thymitis. Death from myasthenia gravis is now rare, as anticholinesterase therapy with pyridostigmine and immunosuppression with steroids or azathioprine have improved muscle

Table 10.5 Osserman classification of myasthenia gravis.	
Group I	Ocular symptoms only
Group IIA	Mild generalized weakness
Group IIB	Moderate bulbar and skeletal symptoms
Group III	Acute severe disease (with respiratory compromise)
Group IV	Chronic severe disease

function for most patients. Thymectomy is often effective in producing an improvement in symptoms, though it is less beneficial to older patients and those with severe myasthenia. Thymomas may become malignant, or grow to a huge size, so resection is often recommended for these reasons alone.

The mainstay of chronic treatment for myasthenia is with a long-acting oral anticholinesterase, usually pyridostigmine. Although rare, an excessive dose of pyridostigmine may precipitate a "cholinergic crisis," with abdominal colic, diarrhea, miosis, lachrimation and excessive salivation. A "myasthenic crisis" results from withdrawal of anticholinesterase therapy, but may also be precipitated by emotion or stress, infection, pregnancy and menstruation. Myasthenic patients learn to manipulate their anticholinesterase medication, and may develop emotional or psychological dependence, becoming fearful if medical staff interfere with treatment. The patients are frequently worried about paralysis in the post-operative period.

Anesthesia for thymectomy in myasthenia

Thymectomy is a major undertaking in a myasthenic patient, and comprehensive pre-operative preparation of the patient, together with communication between surgeon and anesthetist, are important to success. Surgery is best performed while the disease is in remission, but early thymectomy is usually the treatment of choice and excessive delay may result in worsening of myasthenic symptoms. Optimization of anticholinesterase therapy improves muscle function, and plasmapheresis to reduce the concentration of circulating auto-antibodies may be useful in some cases, producing improvement in post-operative respiratory function. Psychological preparation of the patient is important, firstly because stress may precipitate a myasthenic crisis and secondly because the improvement in symptoms following thymectomy is not always immediate, and patients may be disappointed with the result in the early post-operative period.

Pre-operative assessment should include baseline respiratory function tests, and appropriate thoracic imaging as described above for mediastinoscopy. Patients with bulbar muscle involvement may have an impaired cough reflex, leading to tracheobronchial soiling which predisposes to chest infection. Thyroid function should be checked, as there may occasionally be associated thyroid abnormalities. There may also be some myocardial degenerative change associated with myasthenia, and consideration should be given to pre-operative echocardiography. Opinions vary as to the best way to manage anticholinesterase therapy, but on balance it is probably best to continue it on the day of surgery. Patients will be reluctant to omit their pyridostigmine altogether, and post-operative respiratory function will probably be better if it is continued. However, omitting the anticholinesterase may allow avoidance of neuromuscular blocking drugs during surgery.

Thymectomy is usually performed via a median sternotomy, although a limited upper hemisternotomy or a trans-cervical approach (similar to the incision for mediastinoscopy) may also be used. There is little difference in functional outcome between these approaches, although there is less disruption of chest mechanics with the transcervical approach, which may make it easier to avoid prolonged post-operative mechanical ventilation. Median sternotomy is easier for the surgeon and allows for more radical surgery, which is better for large masses or suspected thymoma.

An endobronchial tube is rarely required with any surgical approach for thymectomy. There is little to choose between anesthetic agents, provided the problems associated with myasthenic patients are appreciated. Following induction of anesthesia immediate assisted ventilation may be required, even before neuromuscular blocking drugs are given. In severe myasthenia neuromuscular blocking drugs may be avoided completely, as the muscle-relaxing effect of volatile anesthetics is enhanced. Competitive neuromuscular blocking drugs are not contraindicated in myasthenic patients if used in small doses with adequate monitoring. Suxamethonium is best avoided, though it rarely causes problems, as myasthenic patients are resistant to it and a prolonged phase II block may develop (myasthenic patients do not fasciculate following depolarizing neuromuscular blocking drugs).

Median sternotomy is the least painful approach to major thoracic surgery, but adequate analgesia is vital for effective chest physiotherapy postoperatively. A thoracic epidural is effective in the early post-operative period, but concerns about respiratory depression from opioid analgesia in the presence of neuromuscular disease should not prevent adequate post-operative analgesia. Tracheostomy was routine when thymectomy was first introduced, but in modern practice extubation at the end of the procedure should be the aim. However, this is not always possible and around 50% of patients who have a trans-sternal thymectomy require prolonged mechanical ventilation. Scoring systems have been devised to predict the need for post-operative ventilation, but there is debate about the reliability of these and patients should be considered individually. Severity of disease (Osserman groups III and IV), low forced vital capacity (<15 ml/kg), surgery via median sternotomy, a history of respiratory failure secondary to myasthenia, and pre-operative steroid therapy are all associated with prolonged post-operative ventilation.

Key points

- Patients with mediastinal pathology often have few symptoms at presentation.
- Reliable tissue diagnosis is the key to management of mediastinal masses.
- Mediastinoscopy is potentially a hazardous procedure.
- Effective multidisciplinary management and preparation reduces the risks of thymectomy in myasthenic patients.

FURTHER READING

- Ashbaugh DG. Mediastinoscopy. *Arch Surg* 1970; **100**: 568–73.
- Baraka A. Anaesthesia and myasthenia gravis. *Can J Anaesth* 1992; **39**: 476–86.
- Mackie AM, Watson CB. Anaesthesia and mediastinal masses. *Anaesthesia* 1984; **39**: 899–903.
- Morton JR, Guinn GA. Mediastinoscopy using local anesthesia. *Am J Surg* 1971; **122**: 696–8.
- Osserman KE, Genkins G. Studies in myasthenia gravis – a review of a 20 year experience in over 1200 patients. *Mount Sinai J Med* 1971; **38**: 497–537.
- Vaughan RS. Anaesthesia for mediastinoscopy. *Anaesthesia* 1978; **33**: 195–8.

Chapter 11

Anesthesia for video-assisted thoracoscopic surgery

MAHESH PRABHU

Thoracoscopic inspection of the pleura was first performed under local anesthesia in 1910 by Jacobeaus, a Swedish physician. The inability to illuminate the thoracic space and lack of adequate field of vision held back the development of the technique. The phenomenon of total internal reflection enabled light to be transmitted through a glass fiber and the development of flexible endoscopes. Until the late 1980s thoracoscopic surgery was limited largely to diagnostic techniques. Advances in optical systems, endoscopy equipment and video technology have contributed to increasing the range of video-assisted thoracoscopic surgery (VATS) from diagnostic procedures to more complex therapeutic procedures.

Principles of thoracoscopic surgery

- The minimal requirements for VATS include a rigid telescope, a light source with cable, a camera and an image processor. The optional devices include a slave monitor, a semi-flexible telescope and a video-recorder.
- VATS need higher light output power because blood in the operation field will absorb up to 50% of the light.
- The camera and endoscopic instruments are orientated to face the same way towards the target pathology "baseball diamond concept."

- The access sites should be placed at a sufficient distance from the target pathology to expose a panoramic view and provide room for manipulation.
- The thoracic cage is rigid and the sites of access are limited to the intercostal spaces.
- Single-lung anesthesia is necessary to deflate the lung. Once the lung has collapsed there is no need for insufflation or sealed ports.
- All movement should be under direct vision to prevent any damage to surrounding tissues.
- The operator should be capable of handling any complications and converting to an open procedure if necessary.
- Specific instruments include stapling devices, lasers, dissectors and retractors.

Indications

The common indications for VATS are diagnosis of pleural diseases, cancer staging, management of persistent pneumothorax, retained hemothorax, infected pleural space and collections including empyema, pericardial drainage or window, apical bullectomy and thoracic sympathectomy. Improved technology and growing surgical expertise has led to more procedures being added to the list: thoracic duct ligation, removal of thoracic cyst,

Core Topics in Thoracic Anesthesia, ed. Cait P. Searl and Sameena T. Ahmed. Published by Cambridge University Press.
© Cambridge University Press 2009.

vagotomy, lobar resection and even thymectomy and esophageal surgery.

Contraindications

Pleural symphysis caused by previous thoracic surgery or pleurodesis, bleeding disorders, end-stage pulmonary fibrosis, respiratory insufficiency and hemodynamic instability are some of the contraindications for VATS.

Advantages

Video-assisted thoracoscopic surgery plays a bridging role between the medical and aggressive surgical managements. It is associated with shorter length of hospital stay and less use of pain medication than thoracotomy in the treatment of pneumothorax and minor resections. In the treatment of pneumothorax, VATS is superior to pleural drainage and has a complication profile similar to that for thoracotomy. There is not enough evidence for its use in lobectomies. VATS is associated with better preserved cellular immunity and less inflammatory and immunomodulatory response compared with conventional thoracotomy, which may have an effect on tumor biological behavior.

Pre-operative evaluation

All thoracoscopic surgery should be treated as major procedures because of the pathophysiological changes and the potential for morbidity and mortality. Ambulatory surgery is therefore not appropriate, except for the simplest procedures. A thorough history and physical examination with special attention to the cardiorespiratory status is necessary for all patients. The pre-operative visit is useful to explain the procedure, associated risks, peri-operative care including options for pain relief as well as to provide pre-medication, if necessary. Routine laboratory investigations include full blood count, serum electrolyte levels and electrocardiogram (ECG). Chest radiographs and CT scans help to make a diagnosis and identify potential problems with airway management. Spirometry tests including forced vital capacity (FVC), forced expiratory volume in 1 second (FEV_1) and the ratio FEV_1/FVC provide information about the severity of restrictive or obstructive disease. Pre-operative optimization of respiratory function is achieved by bronchodilators, cessation of smoking, incentive spirometry and physiotherapy.

Intra-operative management

The goals of anesthesia include maintaining stable cardiovascular function, optimizing oxygenation and ventilation, minimizing airway reactivity and preventing ventilatory depression in the postoperative period. The pathophysiological changes of lateral decubitus position, one-lung ventilation, existing disease process and carbon dioxide (CO_2) insufflation must be recognized.

Monitoring: Standard monitoring includes ECG, non-invasive blood pressure measurement, pulse oximetry, capnography, volatile anesthetic agent concentration, temperature and peripheral nerve stimulator. Invasive arterial pressure and central venous pressure monitoring may be needed for patients with poor cardiorespiratory reserve. Monitoring airway pressure, tidal volume and minute volume assist management of ventilation. Pressure-volume loops help in detecting changes in lung compliance and elastance.

Anesthesia: Thoracoscopic surgery has been performed under local, regional or general anesthesia. Pre-medication may include anxiolytics. General anesthesia is usually induced with an intravenous agent such as propofol or thiopentone and maintained with an inhalational agent such as isoflurane in an air/oxygen mixture. Nitrous oxide is preferably avoided because of the risk of expansion in closed air-filled spaces. The inhalational agents provide anesthesia, suppress airway reflexes and induce bronchodilation but have some inhibitory effect on the mechanism of hypoxic pulmonary vaso-constriction (HPV). HPV, a unique autoregulatory mechanism which results in pulmonary vasocon-striction in response to regional alveolar hypoxia ($PaO_2 = 30$ mmHg), is helpful in minimizing the shunt. Total intravenous anesthesia has no effect on HPV. Narcotic analgesia attenuates stress response, reduce minimum alveolar concentration (MAC) requirement of inhalational agents and provide analgesia. Neuromuscular blockade is used to facil-itate endotracheal intubation and maintain muscle relaxation.

Positioning: Most VATS require patient to be placed in a lateral decubitus position with arching of the table to widen the intercostal spaces on the operated side. Care should be taken to prevent dis-placement of the endobronchial tube. Protection of eyes and nerve areas is essential to prevent potential nerve damage. Humidification of anesthetic gases and forced air warming may be used to maintain body temperature.

One-lung ventilation: One-lung ventilation is defined as physiological and anatomical separation of the two lungs by manipulation of the airway. Although thoracoscopic surgery has been consid-ered as a relative indication for one-lung ventila-tion, the onset of complex surgical procedures has justified the need for lung separation. Lung isola-tion may be achieved using either a double-lumen endotracheal tube (DLT), single-lumen endotra-cheal tube with a built-in bronchial blocker (Uni-vent Tube) or an endobronchial blocker such as Arndt (wire-guided) endobronchial blocker or balloon-tipped luminal catheter.

The largest diameter DLT that will pass through the patient's glottis should be used. Smaller tube diameters increase the resistance and the work of breathing. Current practice favors left-sided intuba-tion in the majority of cases. Malposition of DLT is common and position must be confirmed using auscultation techniques and the fiberoptic bron-choscope. Displacement of the tube is manifested by sudden inflation of the non-dependent lung or ventilation difficulty of the dependent lung with increases in airway pressure.

The atelectatic operative lung is fully reinflated and two-lung ventilation is recommened. The bal-loon on the bronchial blocker is deflated and the blocker may be retracted from the bronchus. After discontinuing the inhalational agent and revers-ing muscle relaxation, spontaneous ventilation is resumed. After ensuring adequate oxygenation, ventilation and consciousness, the trachea should be extubated. If the patient is hemodynamically unstable or demonstrates respiratory insufficiency and extubation is not feasible, the double lumen tube should be exchanged for a single lumen endo-tracheal tube.

Analgesia: Post-operative thoracic pain may con-tribute to atelectasis and pulmonary complica-tions by preventing deep respiration and coughing. Pain management strategies include paraceta-mol, NSAIDs, oral opiates, intravenous patient-controlled analgesia, local anesthetic infiltration, intercostal nerve blockade, paravertebral block and even epidural analgesia.

Post-operative care: Routine monitoring of the patient is vital in the recovery room. A portable chest X-ray may be needed to confirm re-expansion of the collapsed lung. Patients should be nursed in upright position and given supplemental oxygen.

Carbon dioxide insufflation

Carbon dioxide gas may be used to insufflate the pleural cavity so as to accelerate lung deflation. Rapid or excessive insufflation of the gas may cause mediastinal shift resulting in hemodynamic insta-bility, bradycardia and hypotension or hypoxia and surgical emphysema. Gas flow is restricted to 2 l/min with the pressure limited to 10 mmHg.

Complications

Video-assisted thoracoscopic surgery is a safe procedure, but extra caution is recommended for patients with a higher risk profile. Factors such as patient age, duration of the VATS procedure, redo-VATS, patients with immune deficiency and conversion to open thoracotomy have been shown to increase the incidence of complications.

Hypoxemia: Arterial hypoxemia, caused by ventilation perfusion mismatch, is treated by increasing inspired oxygen concentration, positive end-expiratory pressure to the ventilated lung, continuous positive airway pressure to the non-ventilated lung and intermittent two-lung ventilation.

Chest pain: The earliest problem is chest pain either in the axillary, scapular or back region. This probably results from thermal damage to the parietal pleura and the periosteum over the ribs.

Respiratory complications: Pre-existing lung disease, lung deflation and pain may encourage sputum retention, decreased functional residual capacity, ventilation perfusion mismatch and atelectasis.

Bleeding: Bleeding may be caused either by injury to blood vessels or by lung perforation. This can be prevented by safe points of entry and electrocoagulation.

Video-assisted thoracoscopic lung resection

Thoracoscopic lobectomy can be oncologically equal to conventional open procedures with an experienced surgeon and have similar survival for early stage non-small cell lung cancer. Peterson *et al.* have demonstrated that thoracoscopic lobectomy is feasible, safe and effective after induction therapy. The advantages compared with a thoracotomy are:
- Shorter length of hospital stay.
- Decreased post-operative pain.
- Preserved pulmonary function.
- Superior cosmetic result.
- Shorter recovery time.

- Improved delivery of adjuvant chemotherapy.
- Lower morbidity in patients with poor lung function.

Relative contraindications to thoracoscopic lobectomy include the inability to achieve complete resection with lobectomy, T3 or T4 tumors, N2 or N3 disease and patients with tumor involving the chest wall. The criterion for tumor size precluding VATS resection has not been defined, although tumors greater than 6 cm in diameter may not be removed without rib spreading.

As thoracoscopic procedures are largely dependent on complete lung isolation, communication between the surgeon and anesthetist is critical. When difficulties with one-lung ventilation are encountered, the surgeon should be aware as soon as possible, so that the problem is managed smoothly and efficiently. If such communication is not established and the operative lung needs to be re-inflated without notice, disaster could result if this coincided with a critical stage of the procedure and can result in bleeding.

The isolation and division of the bronchi and pulmonary blood vessels require more accurate and extensive dissection with VATS than conventional surgery (see Figure 11.1). Thoracoscopic pulmonary resections can be performed by capable surgeons without an increased bleeding risk.

Conversion to thoracotomy

Conversion to a thoracotomy is sometimes required if there is an unexpected change in the patient's condition such as chest wall invasion or the need for a sleeve resection. However, although conversion to thoracotomy should always be considered as a tool available to manage any unexpected situation, conversion rates have been shown to be as low as 1.6–2.5% by McKenna *et al.* in large series by experienced thoracoscopic surgeons. Conversion to an open procedure also becomes necessary

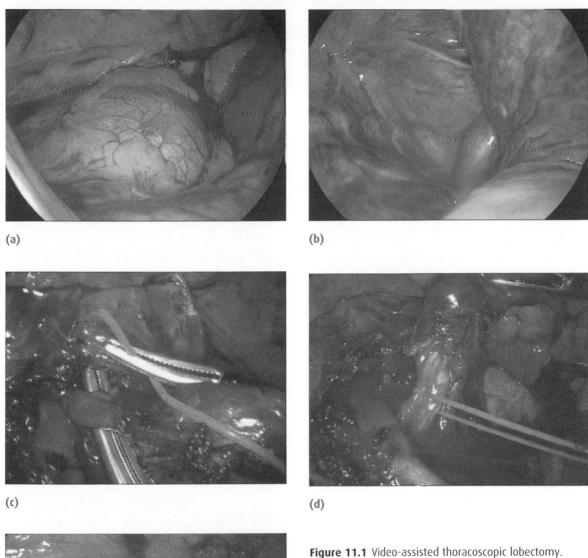

(a)

(b)

(c)

(d)

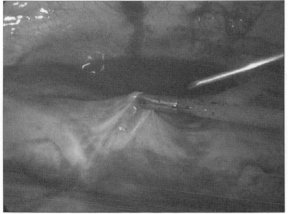

(e)

Figure 11.1 Video-assisted thoracoscopic lobectomy. Following establishment of one-lung ventilation, the ports are placed in the 4th interspace anteriorly, in the 7th interspace (for the camera) and a further one posteriorly. The anatomy is displayed and structures identified starting with the anterior fissure (1a), the main hilar vessels and bronchi and the phrenic nerve (1b: here lying on the SVC). Dissection of the anterior hilum follows with division first of the veins; followed by the bronchial artery (1c) and finally the bronchus (1d). The lymph nodes are sampled and the specimen bagged and removed. Prior to closure a paravertebral catheter is placed, the phrenic nerve is infiltrated (1e) and a drain placed. (*Photographs courtesy of Mr. SA Stamenkovic.*)

if the patient cannot tolerate one-lung ventilation or develops cardiovascular instability.

Conclusion

Video-assisted thoracoscopic surgery has become a vital part of the armamentarium of the surgeon, however, enthusiasm must clearly be tempered with caution; VATS is only a method, rather than the goal of the treatment, and conversion to open procedures should be performed if necessary. There are extra demands on the anesthetist to provide excellent operating conditions whilst ensuring patient safety.

FURTHER READING

- Berry MF, D'Amico T. Complications of thoracoscopic pulmonary resection. *Semin Thorac Cardiovasc Surg* 2003; **19**: 350–4.
- Brodsky JB, Fitzmaurice B. Modern anesthetic techniques for thoracic operations. *World J Surg* 2001; **25**(2): 162–6.
- McKenna RJ Jr, Houck W, Fuller CB. Video-assisted thoracic surgery lobectomy: experience with 1100 cases. *Ann Thorac Surg* 2006; **81**: 421–5.
- Ng CS, Wan S, Hui CW, Lee TW, Underwood MJ, Yim AP. Video-assisted thoracic surgery for early stage lung cancer – can short-term immunological advantages improve long-term survival? *Ann Thorac Cardiovasc Surg* 2006; **12**(5): 308–12.
- Petersen RP, Pham DK, Toloza EM *et al*. Thoracoscopic lobectomy: a safe and effective strategy for patients receiving induction therapy for non-small cell lung cancer. *Ann Thorac Surg* 2006; **82**: 214–19.
- Sedrakyan A, Meulen J, Lewsey J, Treasure T. Video assisted thoracic surgery for treatment of pneumothorax and lung resections: systematic review of randomised clinical trials. *Br Med J* doi:10.1136/bmj.38243.440486.55 (published 22 September 2004).
- Sugi K, Kaneda Y, Esato K. Video-assisted thoracoscopic lobectomy achieves a satisfactory long-term prognosis in patients with clinical stage IA lung cancer. *World J Surg* 2000; **24**: 27–30.

Chapter 12

Anesthesia for lung resection

JOHN JERSTICE

It is important when considering anesthesia for lung resection that the basic principles of anesthesia are not forgotten. A clear and logical approach is needed with careful regard to cardiovascular and pulmonary function.

Appropriate and timely investigations should be performed in order to assess the impact of lung resection on the patient and to guide anesthetic management. It is not the anesthetist's role to say if the patient is "fit enough" for the proposed procedure in the immediate pre-operative period. This should have been considered from the initial surgical referral, with appropriate investigations undertaken and early combined assessment by both surgeon and anesthetist.

The thoracic anesthetist must have a good basic technique with which he or she is completely familiar. However, it is vital that the anesthetist has a full range of techniques at their command as there is rarely ever a completely straightforward thoracic case!

Limited resections: segmental or wedge resections
General considerations

These are very useful surgical techniques facilitating the preservation of lung tissue. These techniques are very good for the excision of benign lesions as

maximum lung is preserved. In malignant disease cure rate is reduced when compared to lobectomy but is still appropriate in patients unfit for "definitive" surgery. These techniques are only possible if the lesion is located in peripheral lung tissue and is well circumscribed.

The surgery can be performed via video-assisted thoracoscopy, a small thoracotomy or standard thoracotomy incision. One-lung ventilation is often useful but not an absolute requirement. A double lumen tube is useful and should be used if possible. I prefer to use a double lumen opposite to the lung to be operated on. As the main bronchi are not being operated on then an argument for the use of a left-sided tube could be made in order to reduce the risk of occlusion of the right upper lobe bronchus.

Monitoring

As the amount of lung tissue lost is small the hemodynamic disturbances are limited to those of the anesthesia alone. Use of invasive monitoring i.e. an A-line is useful but use of a CVP line may not be required unless the patient has a significant history of cardiovascular problems.

Conduct of anesthesia

Anesthesia may be maintained with volatile or total intravenous anesthesia. Short-acting opiates

Core Topics in Thoracic Anesthesia, ed. Cait P. Searl and Sameena T. Ahmed. Published by Cambridge University Press.
© Cambridge University Press 2009.

alfentanil and remifentanil are very useful as they have little post-operative respiratory depression with significant reduction in intra-operative cardiovascular stress. Short-acting muscle relaxants should be used. Atracurium has the advantage of spontaneous degradation especially if an Eaton–Lambert syndrome exists. Normocapnia for the patient or permissive hypercapnia should be the aim to minimize potential barotrauma or volutrauma of the lungs. The use of pressure controlled ventilation is preferred but has the disadvantage that tidal volumes are compliance dependent.

Post-operative considerations

Post-operative analgesia is very important. Good analgesia is crucial so the patient can cough to clear secretions and have good chest expansion to clear CO_2 and avoid hypoxia. Regular prescriptions of paracetamol and a non-steroidal anti-inflammatory should be used with supplementary opiates (a morphine PCA being very useful). The primary analgesic should be a local anesthetic technique, either a thoracic epidural or a paravertebral infusion.

Lobectomy
General considerations

Lobectomy is indicated for malignancy or benign lesions such as bronchiectasis and turberculosis localized to a lobe. The surgery is usually performed through a thoracotomy. Difficulties may arise from tumors invading the chest wall or infections causing pleural thickening or adherence of the lung to the chest wall. The main problems in these situations are increased surgical time, extensive tissue dissection with potentially increased trauma to remaining lung tissue and potential for significant bleeding.

Pre-operative assessment of the patient should follow the usual pattern as outlined in Chapter 4 but with the following extra considerations, especially for patients with infective causes. Careful consideration as to the protection of "good" lung from contamination of infective material is vital. Examination of the chest X-ray, bronchoscopic findings and careful selection of an appropriate endobronchial tube or bronchial blocker should be done well in advance of induction of anesthesia. Use of powerful antibiotics or other anti-microbial agents may have caused significant toxic effects especially on the renal system so assessment of renal function is important. It should be part of the pre-operative assessment to have a high level of concern as to how the patient became infected. For example, is there a history of alcoholism, immunocompromise from drugs or HIV infection?

As with all thoracic surgery it is important to have thought about potential escalation of the procedure proposed and what physiological impact this may have on the patient. An example of this may be a patient scheduled for a right upper lobectomy for a malignancy in whom, once the surgeon has performed the thoracotomy, finds that the tumor cannot be removed by a lobectomy but only a pneumonectomy. The question may be whether the patient has sufficient physiological reserve to survive a pneumonectomy. This should have been considered prior to the start of surgery. Potential problems of bleeding and air leak can be reduced by careful dissection and identification of anatomical structures, the use of stapling devices and fibrin glues.

Monitoring

Intra-operative monitoring should consist of ECG, SaO_2, A-line, capnography and airway pressure monitoring. A CVP should be considered in most cases, especially if an epidural is to be used. The CVP line will guide fluid management and also allow for the use of inotropes if required to maintain BP without need for excessive fluids. Care in positioning the patient is required to prevent pressure areas and nerve damage, whilst allowing the surgeon good operating conditions.

Conduct of anesthesia

Conduct of the anesthesia should be controlled. The use of a benzodiazepine for pre-medication is at the anesthetists' discretion. Anti-sialgogues are best avoided as they may cause the patient difficulty in clearing secretions.

Induction of anesthesia can be with either propofol or thiopentone. Maintenance can be with either a volatile technique or propofol infusion. A short- to medium-acting muscle relaxant can be used. I prefer atracrium in patients with a neoplasm in case an Eaton–Lambert syndrome exists and rocuronium in patients with an infective disease process. Rapid securing of the airway with protection of the healthy lung tissue is vital in patients with an infective pathology where contamination is likely. Neuromuscular blockage monitoring is useful especially at conclusion of the surgery to be sure that full muscle strength had returned before extubation.

Careful controlled ventilation will reduce the risk of barotrauma and volutrauma of the ventilated lung. A pressure control mode of ventilation is preferred with the aim to keep the mean ventilatory pressures as low as possible (less than 22 cm H_2O); peak pressures less than 35 cm H_2O with clearance of CO_2. A degree of permissive hypercapnia is acceptable, the value being dependent on the patient's usual CO_2 level.

At the conclusion of surgery, suctioning of the airway is necessary to remove secretions and debris. Following this, re-inflation of the non-ventilated lung is needed, not only to reverse the atelectasis but also to check for significant air leaks. A pressure of 40 cm H_2O is suggested as sufficient for this purpose. It should be noted that a cough could produce an intrathoracic pressure in excess of 70 cm H_2O! Once the thoracic cavity is closed and airtight with appropriate chest drains connected to underwater seals the patient may be allowed to spontaneously breathe. A check that muscle power has returned is important by use of a peripheral nerve stimulator.

I find that extubation of the patient in the sitting position once they are actively attempting to remove the tube themselves is best.

Post-operative considerations

Good analgesia is crucial. A multimodal method of attack is preferable. Use of regular paracetamol and NSAIDs (if not contraindicated) should supplement a regional local anesthetic technique. A thoracic epidural with low dose levobupivacaine and fentanyl provides excellent analgesia but at the cost of possible hemodynamic instability. The epidural can be run throughout the procedure so reducing the need for large amounts of opiates. Avoiding opiates will prevent depression of respiratory drive and reduce sedation, leading to a patient better able to cough and clear secretions.

A paravertebral infusion has a good analgesic effect with minimal hemodynamic impact. As these are often put in place by the surgeons at the end of surgery they cannot be used to provide intra-operative analgesia. Remifentanil infusions can be used for providing good and effective intra-operative analgesia with no significant post-operative opiate effect if a paravertebral infusion is to be run afterwards.

Pneumonectomy
General considerations

Resection of the entire lung is indicated when lesser lung resection techniques will not provide a curative procedure. Removal of the lung may be indicated if there is massive and persistent hemorrhage, as a completion procedure if lobectomy has not successfully removed the tumor or for extensive infection.

The lung usually is removed through a thoracotomy incision. The hilar structures are dissected, ligated with or without stapling and divided. The main bronchus is divided to leave as short a stump as possible. The bronchial stump is tested, once secretions and blood have been removed by suction, by applying a positive pressure of at least 40 cm H_2O to the airway.

Pre-operative assessment is essentially that for a lobectomy. Extra care needs to be taken in the estimation of remaining post-operative lung function. Loss of functioning lung is the important factor rather than the crude estimation of tissue loss i.e. 55% for a right lung or 45% for a left lung.

Conduct of anesthesia

The use of a double lumen endobronchial tube to the non-operative side is the ideal. This facilitates the protection of the remaining lung from contamination with blood, secretions or infective material from the removed lung and allows for airway toileting once the lung is removed. Other methods of one-lung isolation are on the whole inferior.

With one-lung ventilation, hypoxia is always a potential problem. Early clamping of the main pulmonary artery, thus reducing the shunt, will improve oxygenation. Cardiovascular monitoring is of great importance. An arterial line is useful for accurate and responsive blood pressure monitoring as well as arterial blood gas analysis. A CVP line is very useful in helping with fluid monitoring especially right heart filling pressures. With loss of pulmonary vascular compliance right myocardial function may be compromised and lead to the development of post-pneumonectomy pulmonary edema. Avoidance of excessive crystalloids with the use of colloids or blood has been suggested as a mechanism to reduce the development of pulmonary edema. It cannot be stressed enough that careful management of the ventilation to prevent volu- or barotrauma of the remaining lung is vital. The use of a pulmonary artery catheter cannot be recommended due to difficulty in placing the catheter (it tends to go to the upper lung) and following lung resection inflation of the balloon may be detrimental to myocardial function as even more of the pulmonary vascular bed is occluded.

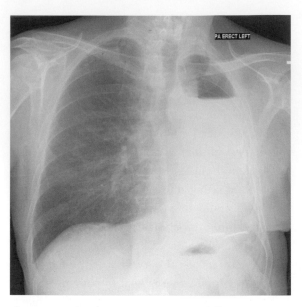

Figure 12.1 The chest X-ray appearance following pneumonectomy.

During the resection of the lung significant arrhythmias may occur due to handling of the hilum and manipulation near the heart. Reduction of venous return due to occlusion of the vena cava may occur. The use of anti-arrhythmic agents may be necessary intra-operatively or post-operatively.

Post-operative considerations

Excellent post-operative analgesia is necessary to optimize the patient's respiratory function. The same techniques as used following lobectomy should be employed. Special care should be taken with fluid balance if epidural analgesia is used. Changes in the ECG may result following surgery if pericarditis occurs; this should not be confused with ischemia. Atrial fibrillation may occur.

Post-operative chest X-ray should demonstrate a central mediastinum with a slowly accumulating fluid level (Figure 12.1). Deviation of the mediastinum may result from herniation of the heart into the pleura space (an acute surgical emergency) or from accumulation of air, fluid or blood. A sudden drop in the fluid level may indicate leakage from the bronchial stump. Development of any of this complication dramatically increases mortality, which is about 5% normally following pneumonectomy.

FURTHER READING

- Alvarez JM, Bairstow BM, Tang C, Newman MA. Post-lung resection pulmonary edema: a case for aggressive management. *J Cardiovasc Vasc Anesth* 1998; **12**(2): 199–205.
- Beck DH, Doepfmer UR, Sinemus C, *et al*. Effects of sevoflurane and propofol on pulmonary shunt fraction during one-lung ventilation for thoracic surgery. *Br J Anaesth* 1998; **86**(1): 38–43.
- Boldt J, Muller M, Uphus D, Padberg W, Hempelmann G. Cardiorespiratory changes in patients undergoing pulmonary resection using different anesthetic management techniques. *J Cardiovasc Vasc Anesth* 2001; **10**(7): 854–9.
- Bolton JW, Weiman DS. Physiology of lung resection. *Clin Chest Med* 1993; **14**(2): 293–303.
- Conacher ID, Velasquez H, Morrice DJ. Endobronchial tubes – a case for re-evaluation. *Anaesthesia* 2006; **61**(6): 587–90.
- Davies RG, Myles PS, Graham JM. A comparison of the analgesic efficacy and side-effects of paravertebral vs epidural blockade for thoracotomy – a systematic review and meta-analysis of randomized trials. *Br J Anaesth* 2006; **96**(4): 418–26.
- Fell SC. Special article: a brief history of pneumonectomy. *Chest Surg Clin N Am* 1999; **12**(3): 541–63.
- Garutti I, Quintana B, Olmedilla L, Cruz A, Barranco M, Garcia de Lucas E. Arterial oxygenation during one-lung ventilation: combined versus general anesthesia. *Anesth Analg* 1999; **88**(3): 494–9.
- Hillier J, Gillbe C. Anaesthesia for lung volume reduction surgery. *Anaesthesia* 2003; **58**(12): 1210–19.
- Mageed NA, El-Ghonaimy YA, Elgamal MA, Hamza U. Acute effects of lobectomy on right ventricular ejection fraction and mixed venous oxygen saturation. *Annals Saudi Med* 2003; **25**(6): 481–5.
- Slinger PD, Johnston MR. Preoperative assessment for pulmonary resection. *J Cardiothorac Vasc Anaesth* 2000; **14**(2): 202–11.

Chapter 13

Surgical treatment options for emphysema

CHRISTOPHER WIGFIELD AND CAIT P. SEARL

Enlargement of air spaces distal to terminal bronchioli with irreversible loss of elastic recoil, results in reduced expiratory airflow and diffuse air trapping. The chest X-ray appearances typically include hyperinflation, barrel chest deformity and hyperlucent lung fields due to parenchymal destruction and bullae formation without fibrosis (Figure 13.1). The alveolar diffusion capacity is reduced and patients present with worsening shortness of breath and progressive exercise limitation. The primary cause of emphysema is cigarette smoking. A minority suffers alveolar-capillary membrane destruction due to alpha$_1$-antitrypsin deficiency, more commonly seen in younger patients with more progressive deterioration of lung functions, particularly FEV$_1$ and T$_L$CO.

No curative interventions are currently available for advanced emphysema. Smoking cessation favorably alters only the rate of decline and infective exacerbations. These are frequently treated with antibiotics and steroid administration. The pharmaceutical mainstay is inhaled bronchodilators. In the absence of curative measures, mucolytics and prophylactic influenza and pneumococcal immunization are advised. Pulmonary rehabilitation may improve exercise tolerance, but many patients eventually require domiciliary oxygen supplementation. Resection of lung parenchyma may appear to be counterintuitive, but consistent improvements of respiratory mechanics and airflow patterns provide a "pulmonic paradox." Surgery for emphysema includes lung volume reduction surgery (LVRS), thoracotomy-based or video-assisted thoracoscopic (VAT) resections and lung transplantation (LTx). Patient selection is paramount for each procedure and both national guidelines (National Institute for Clinical Excellence; NICE) as well as consistent international trial data (NETT trial, International Society for Heart and Lung Transplantation (ISHLT)) are available.

Indications and selection criteria

The indications for surgery in emphysema are predominantly palliative. All surgical options, although essentially superior to medical therapeutics for symptom relief in advanced emphysema, are associated with eventual deterioration of dyspnea in the long term. Few selected patients may experience improved survival. Most patients accepted for LVRS have a FEV$_1$ of 15–40% of predicted and typically elevated TLC and residual volume (RV > 150% of predicted). Persistent hypoxemia (PaO$_2$ < 6 kPa; 45 mmHg) or hypercarbia (PaCO$_2$ > 7.3 kPa; 55 mmHg) are considered adverse factors. Complete smoking cessation for 6 months or more is mandatory. Imaging confirms advanced

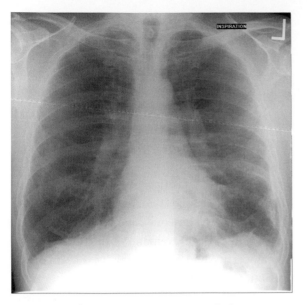

Figure 13.1 Chest X-ray appearance typical of emphysema.

emphysema without fibrotic changes, ideally with heterogenous distribution, i.e. upper lobe predominance. Prohibitive cardiac risk factors must be ruled out. Pulmonary hypertension is seen as multifactorial and correlated with higher operative risk. The NETT trial investigators emphasized the value of pre-operative pulmonary rehabilitation and established subgroups more likely to benefit from LVRS. Marked hypoxemia is typically seen only in end-stage emphysema.

Pre-operative assessment

Candidates for surgery for emphysema require a complete history and examination. The severity of dyspnea and exercise tolerance impairment needs careful evaluation. Advanced spirometry pre- and post-pulmonary rehabilitation and after administration of bronchodilators is performed routinely. Plethysmography provides objective evidence regarding increased residual volumes. A 6-minute walk test gives a useful baseline study to document post-operative improvements. Arterial blood gas analysis (at room air) is helpful for

risk stratification and serology may include alpha-1 antitrypsin and cotinine levels.

After plain chest X-rays, high resolution CT (HRCT) of the thorax and ventilation/perfusion (V/Q) isotope scanning are recommended. Echocardiography provides valvular, ventricular (particularly right) and pulmonary artery pressure evaluation. In borderline candidates cardiopulmonary exercise testing is advocated. The decision to accept a patient for emphysema surgery is also based on absence of relative contraindications – the peri-operative risks are considerable (unadjusted mortality approximately 5%). A BMI of 17–32 is preferable and patients must be well motivated and have realistic expectations in view of their symptomatic benefit. Finally, patients need to be assessed for potential need of lung transplantation.

Surgical options for advanced emphysema

Essentially, three surgical treatment strategies exist for selected subgroups of emphysema patients:
1. Bullectomy.
2. Lung volume reduction surgery (LVRS).
3. Lung transplantation (LTx).

Bullectomy (via thoracotomy or VATs)

A reduction of the thoracic space occupied by hyper-expanded lungs is achieved by selective resection of large emphysematous lung cysts or giant bullae, affecting segments or entire lobes. Surgical stapling devices or lasers are used to resect and seal the least functional lung segments. A variety of approaches are employed according to individual patient situations. Stapling methods and buttressing techniques have evolved to reduce the risk of air leaks. Vigilance is needed when allowing re-expansion of the residual lung. Minimizing air leaks is a primary objective to reduce post-operative morbidity.

Minimally invasive approaches have been advocated with significant advantages in the post-operative period due to improved chest wall physiology compared with open thoracotomies.

The incidence of persistent air leaks, however, has not been shown to be reduced with VAT bullectomy/LVRS. Durable improvement of symptoms after bullectomy is seen only in a select group of patients with giant bullae and well-defined areas of hyperinflation.

Lung volume reduction surgery (LVRS) (via median sternotomy or thoracotomy or VATs)

Formal LVRS comprises a range of pulmonary resection procedures designed to achieve improved gas exchange via volumetric reduction of emphysematous lung. The ideal morphology consists of heterogenous and predominantly upper lobe distribution of severe emphysema, with relatively spared lower zones as frequently associated with aerogenic toxins due to smoking. Improved physiology of the residual lung is thought to occur due to improved expansion of the spared lung areas within the confines of each hemithorax. Proven to be noncontributory to gas exchange the emphysematous lung is stapled and resected. Laser based resections may have higher air leak rates. Video-assisted thoracoscopy or open thoracotomy approaches are also employed. Both approaches have distinct advantages and no single procedure has had superior outcomes. If performed bilaterally, this may be at the same surgery or as staged procedures. The extent and laterality has considerable implications for anesthetic management and need to be determined well in advance. Lung separation is mandatory and double lumen tubes add flexibility, but endobronchial blocker one-lung ventilation may be utilized, particularly for isolated right-sided procedures.

Lung transplantation (LTx) (via thoracotomy, clamshell incisions or median sternotomy)

Lung transplantation is now an established therapeutic option for end-stage emphysema. Patients are assessed according to consensus criteria provided by the ISHLT. Obstructive airway disease and/or emphysema (including alpha1 anti-trypsin deficiency) constitutes 46% of lung transplant procedures, but may not have the same prognostic benefit compared with recipients for cystic fibrosis. Generally, a marked improvement of quality of life is reported, frequently even with selective single lung transplantation.

The primary limitation for LTx is the shortage of suitable allograft donors, and the mortality of advanced emphysema patients on the waiting list is high. Donor evaluation adds to the logistic complexity and unpredictability of this surgical option for emphysema patients. Furthermore, the early mortality risk, although reducing over the last decade, is higher than for the more conservative surgical procedures (15–20% in most units). More recently, LVRS has been proposed as temporary alleviation with a view to later LTx but has not gained widespread acceptance for "bridge to transplantation."

Apart from adverse effects of immunosuppressive regimes and chronic rejection, transplantation also has complex peri-operative implications dependent on utilization of single, single sequential or en bloc implantation. Most frequently, a pneumonectomy is performed of the side shown less contributory on V/Q scans. Lung transplantation for advanced emphysema is currently associated with 81.8% and 48.7% survival at one and five years respectively. For further consideration of lung transplantation see Chapter 13.

Anesthetic and operative considerations
Peri-operative monitoring

Monitoring for LVRS should include 5-lead ECG, pulsoximetry, invasive blood pressure monitoring, a temperature probe and central venous pressure monitoring. Using a Swan–Ganz catheter to assess pulmonary arterial pressure continuously during the procedure may be useful when there are concerns about right ventricular function. With the use of OLV a degree of hypercapnia occurs causing a rise in pulmonary arterial pressure that can cause intra-operative right ventricular decompensation.

Choice of anesthetic agent

In general, short-acting drugs should be used for the maintenance of anesthesia during LVRS to allow the patient to breathe spontaneously as soon as possible following the procedure to decrease the risks of air leakage secondary to positive pressure ventilation. Anesthesia with total intravenous technique using Propofol or using a volatile such as sevoflurane may be preferred to using longer-acting agents. For muscle paralysis, drugs such as vecuronium, rocuronium or cisatracurium might be preferred for both their shorter duration of action and their absence of histamine release.

Anesthetic induction

Pre-oxygenation may need to be for an extended period to achieve denitrogenation. Induction may be associated with hemodynamic instability.

Mechanical ventilation

The aim of ventilation during LVRS is to keep the patient sufficiently oxygenated while also minimizing the risk of air trapping and of causing pneumothorax. The presence of large cystic and bullous areas may induce air progressive trapping and "pulmonary tamponade" physiology resulting in catastrophic reduction of venous return in addition to asphyxia. During ventilation it is important to monitor the volumes being delivered to and exhaled from the lungs to ensure that air is not becoming trapped. This dynamic hyperinflation secondary to positive pressure ventilation per se or aggressive resuscitation attempts may also result in giant bullae forming. As with tension pneumothorax, chest

tube drainage or urgent intra-operative opening of the bullae may be required in this setting.

Analgesia

Pain management post-operatively is best achieved satisfactorily with pre-emptive strategies. These should include either epidural analgesia or paravertebral catheter in addition to patient controlled analgesia (PCA) regimen. Physiotherapy compliance and response is best with adequate analgesia.

Complications associated with LVRS

The risks associated with LVRS are well documented. The main complications include air leaks (up to 45% in one study, generally less than 20% persistent air leaks > 7 days), pneumonia (approximately 10%) and respiratory failure. Persistent air leaks correlate with significant morbidity and require further operative intervention in about 3% of such affected patients. Other complications are related to frequent comorbidities such as thrombotic or ischemic events in a further 5% of patients. For complication details, please refer to the reading list. Overall, the specialist advisors of NICE consider the procedure as beneficial when performed in the setting of multidisciplinary service provision.

Outcomes

There is only historic interest for thoracoplasty procedures, induction of pneumoperitoneum, phrenic nerve palsy and pulmonary denervation in the surgical treatment of emphysema. The selective resection of severely emphysematous lung parenchyma was shown to be beneficial in the 1990s after refining concepts originally described by Brantigan *et al.* The concept of pulmonary "remodeling" found wide acceptance after results of open LVRS were published by Cooper *et al.* in 1994. Different surgical approaches maximize the beneficial effects of enhanced chest wall compliance, improved residual lung function and optimized hemodynamics, particularly RV function.

The evidence for efficacy of LVRS indicates that in appropriately selected candidates, lung function, exercise tolerance and quality of life are markedly improved. These results have been relatively reproducible in various studies and most recently verified in the National Emphysema Treatment Trial (NETT trial). This large-scale prospective randomized controlled trial (>1200 patients) compared surgery with medical therapy and established its superiority. Approximately two-thirds of patients demonstrate improved FEV_1 measurements and similarly 62% recover oxygen independence after LVRS. Variable mortality rates (2.5–23%) were reported and hospital stay ranged widely (10–17 days), mostly dependent on the presence of persistent air leak.

Contraindications

Relative contraindications include the presence of persistent hypoxia or hypercarbia and elevated pulmonary artery pressures (<45 mmHg). Malignancy and systemic disease or cardiac status incompatible with major thoracic surgery needs to be ruled out. Recent high-dose steroid use (>20 mg/day), chronic bronchitis and a significant bronchiectatic element should be absent in candidates. Cigarette dependence or psychosocial issues conflicting with compliance after surgery and during pulmonary rehabilitation need to be addressed well in advance of selection for surgery.

Innovative interventions for advanced emphysema

Endobronchial techniques have been developed and are currently in evaluation. Small devices altering airflow patterns and allowing for reduced air trapping are placed with bronchoscopic access. The distinct advantage of less invasive placement and reduced peri-procedural risk makes these conceptually appealing. These airflow "bypass" devices may be used increasingly as an alternative to surgical approaches. Long-term follow-up data are still lacking for this procedure.

FURTHER READING

- Conacher ID. Anaesthesia for surgery of emphysema: Review Article. *Br J Anaesth* 1997; **79**: 530.
- Cooper JD, Trulock EP, Triantrafilou AN, *et al.* Bilateral pneumonectomy (volume reduction) for chronic obstructive pulmonary disease. *J Thorac Cardiovasc Surg* 1995; **109**:106.
- Fishman A, Martinez F, Naunheim K, *et al.* National Emphysema Treatment Trial Research Group. A randomised trial comparing lung volume reduction surgery with medical therapy for severe emphysema. *N Engl J Med* 2003; **348**: 2059.
- Ginsburg ME. Surgery for emphysema. In Kaiser LR, Kron IR, Spray TL, *et al.*, eds. *Mastery of Cardiothoracic Surgery*, 2nd edn. Philadelphia, PA, Lippincott Williams & Wilkins, 2007.
- NICE guidance: Lung volume reduction surgery for advanced emphysema. 2005. www.nice.org.uk/IP236overview.
- Snell GI. Airway bypass stenting for severe emphysema. http://www.ctsnet.org/sections/thoracic/newtechnoloogy/article-4.html.
- Sukumar MS, Schipper PH, Komanapalli CB, *et al.* Thoracocsopic LVRS. http://www.ctsnet.org/sections/clinicalresources/thoracic/expert
- Ware JH. National emphysema treatment trial – How strong is the evidence? *N Engl J Med* 2003; **348**: 21.
- Young J, Fry-Smith A, Hyde C. Lung volume reduction surgery (LVRS) for chronic obstructive pulmonary disease (COPD) with underlying severe emphysema. *Thorax* 1999; **54**: 779.

Chapter 14

Lung transplantation

CAIT P. SEARL AND STEPHEN CLARK

The lung has historically been the most challenging of the human organs to be successfully transplanted in clinical practice. Since Hardy undertook the first single lung transplant in 1966, the operation has continued to be challenged by the frequent occurrence of bronchiolitis obliterans leading to the progressive onset of respiratory failure in the longer term.

Demographically, the International Society for Heart and Lung Transplantation registry indicates that 78% of recipients in Europe are between 35 and 65 years of age with the majority receiving their transplant for COPD, cystic fibrosis or pulmonary fibrotic disease (Figure 14.1). Only 4.1% were re-transplant procedures, and 77% of recipients were discharged alive from hospital postoperatively. It is possible to transplant lungs singly (SLT) or sequentially as a bilateral lung transplant (BSLT) depending on patient characteristics and the nature of the pathological lung condition present. In some situations combined transplantation of the heart and lungs en bloc is necessary. A bilateral lung transplant is performed where it is clinically necessary to remove all native lung tissue. In the context of chronic lung sepsis in cystic fibrosis or bronchiectasis, single lung transplantation would fail as infection may cross-contaminate from the native remaining lung into the graft.

Similarly, extensive destruction of both lungs in emphysema may suggest the need for bilateral replacement to avoid air trapping in a remaining overly compliant native lung, resulting in mediastinal shift and compromise of the contralateral graft. A single lung transplant is an attractive approach to the treatment of lung failure. The operation can often be performed without the acute lung injury and other attendant risks associated with cardiopulmonary bypass. There is an economy in the use of scarce donor organs with two lung recipients benefiting from each donor and, in the event of acute or chronic injury to the graft, some viable native lung tissue will remain. Fibrotic lung conditions with normal pulmonary vasculature, a relatively immobile mediastinum and no native overinflation are most suited to this type of pulmonary transplant procedure (Figures 14.2a, b). However, SLT is used with varying enthusiasm between centers for selected patients with emphysema (with or without alpha$_1$-antitrypsin deficiency) and sarcoidosis.

A controversial area is lung transplantation for primary pulmonary hypertension. Here, in the absence of structural injury to the heart, bilateral lung transplantation may suffice though many centers still advocate combined heart and lung transplantation. Some centers are performing SLT alone

Core Topics in Thoracic Anesthesia, ed. Cait P. Searl and Sameena T. Ahmed. Published by Cambridge University Press.
© Cambridge University Press 2009.

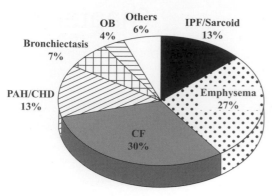

Figure 14.1 Transplant recipient diagnoses. PAH/CHD, pulmonary arterial hypertension/congenital heart disease; OB, obliterative broncholitis; CF, cystic fibrosis; IPF, idiopathic pulmonary fibrosis.

in these circumstances. Survival for all three modalities of treatment for primary pulmonary hypertension is similar. Transplantation of both lungs enbloc with the heart for pulmonary pathology is becoming less popular although this was the early means of lung replacement. Some centers still use this approach in circumstances where total lung replacement is required (the same indications as for BSLT). Although at first sight this may seem wasteful of scarce donor hearts where sequential lung transplantation will suffice, the structurally normal recipient heart is harvested and used for a heart transplant candidate (the "domino" operation).

Lung recipient assessment and selection

Lung transplant assessment tests will typically also include sputum tests for *Aspergillus* and *Aspergillus* precipitins. A 6-minute walk test is performed which measures the distance a patient is able to walk in a given time and the degree of arterial desaturation that results during this exertion. Not only does this give a measure of symptomatic restriction but it also has prognostic value. Values of less than 300 m are seen in patients in end-stage pulmonary failure. Computerized tomography (CT) is used to study the texture of lung parenchyma and

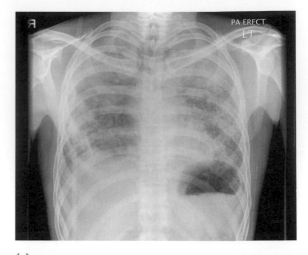

(a)

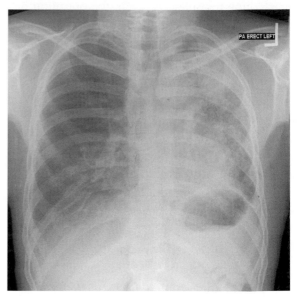

(b)

Figure 14.2 Chest X-rays showing fibrotic lung disease (a) pre-transplant and (b) post single lung transplant.

identify areas of maximal lung destruction or bullous disease accurately. This, along with the results of ventilation-perfusion scanning assists with the decision of whether to perform BSLT or SLT in those conditions where either might be considered and, if SLT is selected, which side should be transplanted. For SLT it is usual to replace the lung with poorer perfusion. It is always preferable to explant a lung if there is evidence of chronic sepsis within it or if a bullus that is likely to rupture is present. These investigations also help to identify those emphysematous patients who might be suitable for lung volume reduction surgery as an alternative to transplantation with the aim of improving their ventilatory mechanics with symptomatic relief.

Detailed microbiological screening is an essential part of the assessment with attention also paid to cultures performed over the preceding months and years at the referring center. This information identifies patients likely to be colonized with multiply resistant organisms (especially pseudomonads in the cystic population) and helps direct antibiotic prophylaxis in the peri-operative period. Of late the particular importance of colonization with *Burkholdaria cepacia* has been recognized as an important predictor of post-transplant mortality which may influence acceptance or post-operative management. In the cystic patient population with chronic sepsis and malabsorption, a nutritional assessment is vital since wound healing is impaired and the loss of muscle bulk may result in insufficient respiratory effort to permit weaning from the ventilator in the post-operative period.

Cardiopulmonary bypass is used routinely for BSLT and in about 20% of cases undergoing SLT, so coincidental cardiac disease must be identified. Older patients and those with relevant risk profiles undergo cardiac catheterization with coronary angiography. Right heart catheterization is undertaken in patients considered for lung transplantation for pulmonary hypertension. This can be supplemented by pulmonary angiography if pulmonary thromboendarterectomy might be considered as an alternative to transplantation. The remainder of the assessment is designed to identify contraindications to organ replacement. Absolute contraindications to pulmonary transplantation might include multi-organ failure and ongoing sepsis. Current malignancy, active peptic ulceration and inadequate conventional ther-

apy are also important. Relative contraindications include peripheral and cerebral vascular disease, diabetes, obesity, osteoporosis and ischemic heart disease. On occasion patients who have acute pulmonary failure (for example, ARDS) and are ventilator-dependent are referred to be considered for transplantation. Pulmonary transplantation is seldom successful under these circumstances as sepsis and multiorgan failure are common. However, if attempted, it is worth considering single lung replacement since the potential for recovery in the native lung is present in many cases of acute respiratory disease.

Lung donor criteria and selection

Specific considerations for lung donation must include a demonstration of good gas exchange with no evidence of aspiration, embolism or pneumonia. Smokers and patients with a history of mild asthma may still be considered as potential lung donors. In practice, only a minority of multiorgan donors are suitable for lung donation as potential lung injury may arise in a number of ways including trauma, aspiration and pulmonary edema. Examination of the chest radiograph is essential. Aspirates taken from the endotracheal tube should be examined microscopically and Gram stained at the donor hospital. Mixed Gram negative and positive organisms and numerous polymorphs in the aspirate may indicate potentially unacceptable infection. Previous culture results should be requested and considered. Flexible bronchoscopy can be useful to facilitate full expansion of the lungs and obtain good specimens of pulmonary secretions. Lung function is assessed by gas exchange. A useful standardized measure is the PaO_2 with the donor ventilated on 100% oxygen and with 5 mmHg of positive end-expiratory pressure to optimize ventilation. A value of less than 35 kPa is an indicator of significant lung injury and many centers will not use lungs where a value of less than 50 kPa is recorded. The aspiration of blood from individual upper and lower lobe pulmonary veins is often useful when evaluating single lungs where 45 kPa is a reasonable level of acceptability. Final assessment of the lungs is performed by the donor surgeon, who can see bullae and traumatized lung and feel areas of consolidation. Edematous lungs feel heavy and spongy and may lead the donor team to reject the organs for use.

Lung recipient–donor matching

Matching of donor and recipient for lung transplantation is largely a crude process focusing on blood group and dimensions with no prospective match for tissue type. Size can be assessed in a number of ways including comparison of measurements taken from donor and recipient chest radiographs. Donor and recipient heights are a useful guide to matching, with a 10–15% mismatch permissible. However, it is now generally recognized that donors should be matched to the predicted lung size of the recipient rather than the pathological size since thoracic capacity and chest wall mechanics will normalize after transplantation. Cytomegalovirus status is an important consideration. Cytomegalovirus mismatch here has greater implications for a lung recipient in the event of seroconversion or re-activation in the grafted tissue.

Lung retrieval and preservation

The thoracic organs are retrieved through a median sternotomy. When the aorta is cross-clamped and the heart cardiopleged, infusion of preservative into the lungs can proceed through the pulmonary artery catheter. Simultaneous topical cooling of heart and lungs with cold saline solution proceeds throughout this time. Pulmonary preservative solutions exist in many forms. Traditionally Euro–Collins solution has been used, which is essentially an intracellular fluid. Recently other preservatives based on extracellular fluids have been used such as Perfadex (low potassium dextran) with more encouraging results and the potential to extend organ ischemic times. Prostaglandins may help prevent leukocyte sequestration and also optimize perfusion of the pulmonary capillary bed and are given before infusion of the pulmoplegic solution. Preservation is achieved by cooling with extracorporeal circulation in some centers but most units use a hypothermic cold flush perfusion technique. Ischemic times of 6–8 h can be safely achieved. The anesthetist is now asked to ventilate the lungs by hand with air to prevent alveolar collapse. Occasional cessation of ventilation will facilitate excision of the bloc, which is undertaken when cardioplegia and pulmonary preservative solutions have both been given. The anesthetist is now asked to withdraw the endotracheal tube into the upper trachea whilst still ventilating. A clamp can now be placed across the trachea below the endotracheal tube and the trachea divided above. All that remains is to divide the connective tissue behind the ascending aorta and trachea and remove the entire heart–lung bloc. The trachea is stapled to allow removal of the clamp whilst leaving the lungs inflated for transfer.

Anesthesia for single lung transplantation

By the time of transplant, the recipient's pathophysiology is likely to show:

- Restrictive pattern of respiratory failure.
- Minimal reserve.
- Impaired diffusion capacity.
- Significant A-a gradient.
- Moderate pulmonary hypertension at least.
- Variable degrees of right heart dysfunction.

The operation of single lung transplantation is effectively at start a pneumonectomy in a patient who under normal circumstances would be judged unfit for such an operation. Pre-operatively patients are usually given antibiotics as per the microbiologists' advice and immunosuppressive agents such as cyclosporin and azathioprine. Sedative premedication is usually avoided.

The aim of induction is to maintain hemodynamic stability and oxygenation of the patient through commencement of anesthesia. No induction agent has ever been shown to be better than another for this purpose. At the Freeman hospital, all the consultants use a range of induction agents, usually the same as they would employ for their regular lists. A double lumen tube appropriately sided and sized is used – Robertshaw DLTs are most commonly utilized here. The opposite sided tube to the operative side is employed. Other means necessary to isolate lung (bronchial blockers etc.) may also be used and are available when necessary. The tube position is checked by standard regimes including a bronchoscope if necessary.

The patient is positioned in the lateral position for thoracotomy, with the groins prepared and partially exposed to allow for rapid positioning of cardiopulmonary bypass cannula in the femoral vessels. Maintenance of anesthesia is as standard for thoracotomy with either volatile or total intravenous anesthesia. While there are theoretical relative contraindications to the use of volatiles (abolition of hypoxic pulmonary vasoconstriction), these probably do not apply in diseased lungs. There is no proven benefit to using propofol TIVA. Air/oxygen mixes are used for ventilation. The use of nitrous oxide is avoided because of the risks of increasing pulmonary vascular resistance, expanding bullae, etc. A lateral thoracotomy is performed and the native lung is excised with ligation of inferior and superior pulmonary veins and pulmonary artery. The bronchus is divided and the native organ removed. Care is taken not to contaminate the pleural space with endobronchial secretions. Meticulous hemostasis at the hilum is established. The donor lung is now prepared by trimming the left atrial cuff, cutting the pulmonary artery to length and excising the stapled end of the bronchus to deflate the lung. Implantation commences with the bronchial anastomosis followed by the left atrial anastomosis with the clamp left applied. The pulmonary artery anas-

tomosis is performed in the same fashion and the donor organ is now de-aired by partially releasing the clamp from the pulmonary artery and de-airing through the left atrial anastomosis. The left atrial clamp can now be removed. Ventilation of the new lung commences. Apical and basal chest drains are inserted.

Intra-operative problems are divisible into three main categories:

- One-lung anesthesia.
- Clamping of the pulmonary artery prior to pneumonectomy.
- Donor lung reperfusion.

Problems with one-lung anesthesia

These are associated with the presence of a large shunt, a low PaO_2 and CO_2 retention. These all may be associated with cardiovascular instability. Management is similar to management of one-lung anesthesia in any situation:

- Increase FiO_2.
- Alter ventilatory pattern (I:E ratios, volumes).
- Oxygen insufflation/recruitment maneuvers.
- Intermittent disconnection, particularly if breath stacking is occurring.

Oxygenation often improves with time and also may do so with clamping of the pulmonary artery. If the patient is too unstable for one-lung anesthesia to remain sustainable, cardiopulmonary bypass is a sensible alternative. Making this decision early is probably prognostically better for both patient and anesthetist!

Pulmonary artery clamping

When the contralateral PA is clamped there is inevitably a sudden increase in pressure in the remaining PA. This may precipitate right heart failure, particularly in a patient who is already relatively cardiovascularly compromised. At this stage inotropic support may become necessary and should be directed particularly at supporting the right heart, e.g. milrinone, isoprenaline. Again, cardiopulmonary bypass should be considered before the situation becomes irretrievable.

Donor lung reperfusion

If the vascular anastamosis is achieved before a satisfactory bronchial one, a large shunt is provoked – usually a short-lived problem.

At the end of the procedure the double lumen tube is changed to a single lumen endotracheal tube to allow a period of post-operative ventilation on intensive care. Analgesia is managed with a combination of paravertebral/epidural block and an intravenous opiate via a patient-controlled analgesia device or infusion. Usually the earlier a lung transplant recipient is extubated the better.

Anesthesia for sequential bilateral lung transplantation

At many centers, this procedure is undertaken as sequential single lung transplants to avoid the perceived increase in acute lung injury post-operatively which is said to accompany extracorporeal perfusion. In our institution, all sequential bilateral lung transplants are done with cardiopulmonary bypass support with little evidence of additional lung injury. The problems are mainly associated with separation from bypass in patients whose hearts have just withstood 4–6 hours of cardiopulmonary bypass.

The operation is approached through a submammary "clam shell" incision which divides the sternum transversely. A median sternotomy is a less painful incision which can be used in some cases though access can sometimes be more of a challenge. The patient is fully heparinized, the pericardium is opened and the patient is placed on cardiopulmonary bypass with an ascending aortic inflow cannula and venous drainage from individual cannulation of the caval veins. Care is taken to preserve the phrenic nerve while mobilizing structures at each hilum especially in patients with septic

lung disease where large lymph nodes and dense hilar adhesions make excision of the lung difficult. Excision of each lung proceeds in turn and in cases of pulmonary sepsis, the pleural cavities are irrigated thoroughly with the antiseptic Taurolin. Implantation of the donor lungs is performed in exactly the fashion described for single lung transplantation, the right side being anastomosed first. The patient is usually cooled to 32 °C during implantation, the heart being allowed to continue to beat and eject in sinus rhythm. After implantation, de-airing and reperfusion are performed and ventilation is recommenced. At normothermia cardiopulmonary bypass can be weaned. It is important that the pulmonary artery pressure at reperfusion is controlled. A number of experimental studies have shown reduced lung reperfusion injury when this is the case and even a short period of controlled pressure reperfusion is beneficial. We keep the mean PA pressure at less than 20 mmHg for at least 10 minutes while reperfusing a lung transplant. Each thoracic cavity is drained with basal and apical drains and the wound is closed. The patient is then returned to the intensive care unit for further monitoring and can usually be extubated at 8–12 hours post-operatively. Epidural analgesia is essential following the "clam shell" incision. Return to the ward is usually at about 24–48 hours.

Elsewhere, where the preferred manner is sequential lung transplantation via bilateral thoracotomies, anesthesia is more challenging with the changing of double lumen tube and patient position halfway as well as all the problems and more of single lung transplantation anesthesia. With bilateral thoracotomies, analgesia remains a major issue with the standard remaining epidural.

Peri- and post-operative care for lung transplants

On notification of a possible donor the selected recipient is admitted and reassessed for deterioration or unexpected infection. Infection and colonization of the airway and lung is a major feature of lung transplant and a leading cause of morbidity and mortality in the post-operative period. Antibiotic prophylaxis is largely directed by the known flora of the recipient but flucloxacillin is used for Gram positive cover and metronidazole for Gram-negative cover in the absence of other positive cultures. Colomycin is administered by nebulizer in the immediate post-operative period. Antibiotic therapy is modified in the first few days after transplant as the results of peri-operative donor and recipient bronchoalveolar lavages become available. In the absence of infection, antibacterial agents are stopped after the first routine bronchoscopy and biopsy at one week provided airway anastomoses appear healthy. Aciclovir, antifungal agents and pneumocystis prophylaxis are routinely used.

Immunosuppression commences pre-operatively with the administration of azathioprine and cyclosporin A. Methylprednisolone is administered at reperfusion and continued intravenously for 24 h after which oral steroids may be commenced. However, since many pulmonary recipients have malabsorption and early cyclosporin levels may be erratic, antithymocyte globulin (ATG) may be administered for the first 3 days as induction therapy, with dosage and timing being regulated by daily flow cytometry lymphocyte counts. In recent years, other immunosuppressants have been put forward for use in post-operative immunosuppressive regimens. In particular, the use of induction therapy with ATG has been questioned due to concerns over increased rates of infection and of post-transplant lymphoma, though this is very controversial. Tacrolimus (FK506), mycofenalate mofetil (MMF) and rapamycin have been investigated but so far no conclusive advantages have been demonstrated although side-effect profiles may be subject to some improvements.

If any lung injury is present in the immediate post-operative period, ventilation can present great difficulties. Such reperfusion injury results from the sequestration of neutrophils in the lung parenchyma with release of injurious enzymes and oxygen free radicals. Lungs may be edematous or infected with poor gas exchange. Meticulous control of fluid balance, optimization of ventilation and microbiological control are needed in this situation. Nitric oxide administration has many benefits in reperfusion injury and is distributed preferentially to ventilated areas of the lung. It improves ventilation-perfusion matching and lowers pulmonary artery pressures. It reduces the adhesion of neutrophils to the endothelium and so alleviates reperfusion injury. A number of other interventions (controlled pressure reperfusion, pentoxifylline, extracorporeal filters, adhesion molecule modulators) affecting neutrophil sequestration in the lung have been put forward to try to combat this problem post-operatively but have not been widely evaluated in clinical practice.

In the case of the single lung transplant for emphysema, the residual emphysematous over-compliant lung can inflate excessively, with air trapping and resultant mediastinal shift if the expiratory period of ventilation is insufficient. Modification of the ventilatory cycle can help but sometimes it is necessary to use independent ventilation of each lung through a double lumen endotracheal tube.

Transbronchial biopsy and bronchoalveolar lavage with a flexible bronchoscope under sedation is performed at one week, one month and then every three months before reverting to annual biopsies to detect rejection and direct antimicrobial intervention. Additional biopsies are taken if rejection is suspected on the grounds of unexplained fever, symptomatic deterioration with arterial desaturation or a fall in pulmonary function tests including spirometry and transfer factor.

Outcomes and complications of lung transplantation

Generally, 30-day survival is approximately 85%, with 75% surviving to one year. At 5 years, 45% remain alive and 25% after a decade. Survival curves for bilateral lung transplantation are a little better than for unilateral procedures. The early decline in survival mirrors that seen in heart transplantation and reflects operative mortality and donor organ dysfunction. The causes of peri-operative mortality include unsuspected donor lung injury (infection, edema, embolic disease or poor preservation) and reperfusion injury. Specific technical difficulties include anastomotic stenoses with pulmonary oligemia (pulmonary arterial obstruction) or pulmonary edema (venous stenosis) and airway ischemia and dehiscence with resultant mediastinitis. The vascular supply of bronchial and tracheal anastomoses is compromised and early dehiscence with ischemia is a life-threatening complication with prolonged air leak and mediastinitis. Attention to detail when the anastomosis is performed with care not to denude the airway minimizes this risk. It is no longer thought necessary to wrap the anastomosis in a vascularized pedicle or omentum. Concurrent steroid therapy (once considered a contraindication to lung transplantation) may even reduce dehiscence as development of capillaries at the anastomosis is enhanced. Some early in-hospital deaths result from infection and acute rejection episodes.

Quality of life is significantly improved by transplantation for pulmonary failure. Studies in lung transplant patient groups consistently show improvements in functional status and the perception of symptoms, irrespective of the type of transplant performed or the primary pathology.

FURTHER READING

- Aris RM, Routh JC, Lipuma JJ, *et al.* Lung transplantation for cystic fibrosis patients with *Burkholderia cepacia* complex. Survival linked to genomovar type. *Am J Respir Crit Care Med* 2001; **164(11)**: 2102–6.
- Aziz TM, El-Gamel A, Saad RG, *et al.* Pulmonary vein gas analysis for assessing donor lung function. *Ann Thorac Surg* 2002; **73(5)**: 1599–604; discussion 1604–5.
- Charman SC, Sharples LD, McNeil KD, *et al.* Assessment of survival benefit after lung transplantation by patient diagnosis. *J Heart Lung Transplant* 2002; **21(2)**: 226–32.
- Clark SC, Sundershan C, Khanna R, *et al.* Controlled reperfusion and pentoxifylline modulate reperfusion injury after single lung transplantation. *J Thorac Cardiovasc Surg* 1998; **115(6)**: 1335–41.
- Hardy JD, Alican F. Lung transplantation. *Adv Surg* 1966; **2**: 235–64.
- Szeto WY, Kreisel D, Karakousis GC, *et al.* Cardiopulmonary bypass for bilateral sequential lung transplantation in patients with chronic obstructive pulmonary disease without adverse effect on lung function or clinical outcome. *J Thorac Cardiovasc Surg* 2002; **124(2)**: 241–9.

Chapter 15

Anesthesia for pulmonary endarterectomy

KAMEN VALCHANOV AND ALAIN VUYLSTEKE

The vast majority of patients surviving a pulmonary embolism will dissolve their embolic thrombus and continue to lead an unrestricted life. However, up to 4% of them will develop an organized clot inside the pulmonary artery. This organized clot will progressively transform or evolve in a neo-formation that will end up obstructing the pulmonary artery and cause pulmonary hypertension (referred to as chronic thromboembolic pulmonary hypertension or CTEPH). This will in turn lead progressively to right heart failure.

At present, pulmonary endarterectomy (PEA – previously known as pulmonary thrombo-endarterectomy or PTE) is the only curative option for a subgroup of patients suffering from CTEPH. The aim of this chapter is to summarize current knowledge about CTEPH and discuss the perioperative and anesthetic management of patients scheduled for PEA.

Chronic thromboembolic pulmonary hypertension

Patients of different gender and age will usually present with symptoms such as dyspnea, reduced exercise tolerance, fatigue, syncope and/or angina-like chest pain. Only half of these patients will recall a past episode of deep venous thrombosis or pulmonary embolism, and many will have gone through a symptom-free period after the original thromboembolic episode. It is noteworthy that up to 50% of patients have no past medical history of significance; and CTEPH may be in these cases the result of asymptomatic thromboembolic episodes.

Pathophysiology

The mechanisms behind the development of the disease are not clearly understood but it has been shown that it is not solely the result of in situ thrombosis in the pulmonary arteries. Approximately half of the patients exhibit known thrombotic tendencies like protein-C deficiency, factor V Leiden deficiency, anti-phospholipid syndrome or other autoimmune disorders; and in situ thrombosis in CTEPH may be initiated or aggravated by abnormalities in the clotting cascade, endothelial cells or platelets, all of which interact in the coagulation process. Various molecules are involved, including endothelin, plasma monocytes chemo-attractant protein-1, IL-6, IL-10 and TNF-α. On histological examination thickenings of the pulmonary vessels that can be seen protruding in the vascular lumen appear eccentric and contain septa and webs. Smooth muscle proliferation in the pulmonary vessel wall is observed most of the time.

Core Topics in Thoracic Anesthesia, ed. Cait P. Searl and Sameena T. Ahmed. Published by Cambridge University Press.
© Cambridge University Press 2009.

Classification

Pulmonary hypertension was classified by the World Health Organization in 1998 into five categories, with CTEPH being category four (see Chapter 4).

Prognosis

Survival is directly related to the mean pulmonary arterial pressure (MPAP) at the time of diagnosis and approximately 90% of patients presenting with an MPAP above 50 mmHg will die within 5 years of diagnosis. Medical therapy can only alleviate the symptoms but will not, at present, stop the progress of the disease. Pulmonary endarterectomy is the only therapeutic option for these patients but incurs a generally accepted quoted peri-operative mortality of 10%. Mortality is lower in centers operating routinely on many patients.

Diagnosis

The diagnosis is often delayed or unrecognized because signs are often subtle in the beginning. Clinical examination can reveal signs of right heart failure or tricuspid regurgitation such as high jugular pressure and hepatomegaly. Peripheral and central cyanosis is classical at later stages. Chest auscultation can reveal an accentuated second heart sound and a distinctive murmur over the pericardium and lung fields. Some patients will rapidly become wheelchair bound as they are unable to make the slightest physical effort.

Electrocardiogram changes are often non-specific and show right ventricular hypertrophy and right axis deviation.

Trans-thoracic echocardiography is a non-invasive investigation to assess the function of the right heart and estimate pulmonary artery pressures. It reveals right heart chambers' enlargement, tricuspid regurgitation as well as leftward displacement of the septum. Transesophageal echocar-

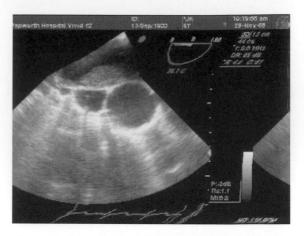

Figure 15.1 Transesophageal echocardiography still image showing an organized thrombus in the right pulmonary artery.

diography (TOE), usually performed in the peri-operative period, will be useful to evaluate the presence of an ASD, intracardiac thrombi and even sometimes the organized thrombus in the main pulmonary arteries (Figure 15.1).

Right heart catheterization allows direct measurement of pulmonary arterial and right ventricular pressures, as well as cardiac output.

Radioisotope scanning can illustrate the mismatched lung segments and exact location of perfusion defects. Computerized tomography scanning with pulmonary angiography is a useful tool in distinguishing between proximal and distal disease. High-resolution spiral CT with contrast is useful, demonstrating mosaic perfusion of both lung fields, and permitting visualization of the pulmonary vascular tree. Angioscopy can be performed pre-operatively to confirm operability in patients with equivocal indications from angiography. Magnetic resonance imaging (MRI) can provide further three-dimensional anatomical information, but is not as accurate as pulmonary angiography in determining the extent and distribution of the disease. Coronary angiography should be performed to assess the need for bypass grafting in the presence of known risk factors.

Routine blood tests, including coagulation screening and arterial blood gas analysis are mandatory. Lung function tests are used to exclude pulmonary parenchymal disease.

Duplex scanning of the legs can reveal scarring from previous thrombosis.

Treatment

To date, no medical therapy has proven curative in cases of CTEPH and only surgery can result in a complete clearance of the pulmonary vascular tree, subsequent remission of clinical symptoms and a dramatic improvement in quality and length of life. Lung transplantation has been offered for many years, but the scarcity of donor organs, the prospect of lifelong immunosuppression and the lower survival at 5 years, make it an unrealistic and uneconomical option for those patients amenable to conventional PEA. Angioplasty of the pulmonary artery with inflatable balloon has been reported in a small number of patients.

Medical treatment consists largely of pulmonary vasodilators like the phosphodiesterase type-5 inhibitor sildenafil, the endothelin-antagonist bosentan or prostacyclin analogs such as iloprost. It is accepted that these patients should be anticoagulated and will benefit from a filter in the inferior vena cava. Medical treatment can be used as a bridge to the operation, or to palliate symptoms when surgery is deemed futile.

Pulmonary endarterectomy (PEA)

The surgical treatment of chronic thromboembolic pulmonary hypertension was first described by Daily in 1980. In 2005, at least six centers in the world were performing this operation routinely. Pulmonary endarterectomy is a definitive treatment for CTEPH and involves removal of the organized embolic material from both pulmonary arteries.

Patient selection

Only disease limited to main, lobar and proximal segmental arteries is amenable to the surgical treatment. The main pre-operative challenge remains in separating those patients with central disease from the ones with exclusively peripheral disease. Moreover, involvement of small vessels is a poor predictive indicator, as a surgical central clearance may not decrease substantially MPAP and right ventricular stress. In experienced hands and absence of peripheral pulmonary vascular disease, the risk of peri-operative death relates more to the degree of pre-operative heart failure than to intra-operative factors. Apart from these disease-specific factors, it is important to ensure that any other comorbidity is well controlled, as it will add to the insult of surgery and cardiopulmonary bypass (CPB), and prolong post-operative recovery. In some cases, these may also be a contraindication to surgery.

Surgical technique

The surgical approach is usually through a median sternotomy and involves use of CPB. Other approaches such as thoracotomies have been attempted with no success. Bicaval cannulation is advantageous as it offers an unobstructed view of the pulmonary arteries and adequate drainage from the head vessels.

An increased collateral blood flow to the lungs is observed in these patients, rendering visualization of the pulmonary arteries difficult even after aortic cross-clamping. It is therefore advocated that deep hypothermic circulatory arrest (DHCA) must be used in all patients. Alternative strategies such as antegrade perfusion and balloon occlusion of the bronchial arteries have been proposed but so far not proven superior in relation to surgical success and patient's outcome.

The technique used for DHCA is often specific to each cardiac center and will often involve administration of thiopentone, steroids, phenytoin, mannitol or other agents with alleged or demonstrated neuroprotection abilities. It is unknown if any of those agents affect the reperfusion insults in the brain, lungs or other organs. Surface cooling with head ice packs and heart cooling devices are also used.

The disease is always bilateral and right and left endarterectomies are performed sequentially. The surgical planes are sometimes difficult to find. Intraoperative use of an angioscope to assist the dissection and evaluate the vascular clearance has been advocated.

Additional surgery, such as ASD closure, coronary grafting or valve surgery is usually performed during rewarming, after completion of the endarterectomy. Some argue not to repair an existing small ASD defect, which may act as a natural vent in case of elevated right-sided pressure.

Clamping of the aorta and cardioplegia are routinely required for cardiac protection, and topical cooling of the heart (with a cooling blanket) has proven useful. Division of SVC may help achieve better visualization of the surgical field and the left heart is commonly vented through the superior pulmonary vein.

Throughout the intervention, the patients require vascular access for the administration of drugs, and invasive pressure monitoring, including pulmonary artery pressure. The surgeon usually replaces the pulmonary artery catheter after the dissection, and great care in mobilizing it should ensue to avoid traumatic rupture of the pulmonary vessels. The catheter should not be moved or wedged to measure capillary pressure (we usually use a default pulmonary capillary wedge pressure of 10 mmHg for hemodynamic calculations).

Patients must continue their anticoagulation to the day of the operation, usually with a vitamin K inhibitor. Administration of vitamin K on induction of anesthesia will usually have reversed the effect by the time the patient's chest is closed. Anticoagulation management during CPB with heparin is commonly used, and protamine used to reverse its effect after separation from CPB. Recombinant-hirudin has been used in patients with HIT. Some centers administer antifibrinolytics routinely in those patients.

A cell saver should be used throughout the procedure, and with the exception of concentrated red cells, it is uncommon to transfuse platelets concentrates or fresh frozen plasma at any stage. Centers operating on many patients routinely use human albumin 4.5% as the main resuscitation fluid, including in the prime of CPB circuits.

Anesthetic management

The peri-operative management of patients undergoing pulmonary endarterectomy is complex and involves a multidisciplinary team of physicians, surgeons, anesthetists and intensivists. Thorough pre-operative investigation and ascertaining the appropriateness of surgery is essential.

PRE-MEDICATION

Sedative pre-medication with opioids or benzodiazepines may be used, but care must taken to ensure that the patient is neither hypoxic nor hypercarbic as this would increase pulmonary vascular resistance. Some centers prefer not to use premedication and rely on good pre-operative counselling by the anesthetist and surgical team.

MONITORING

In addition to the routine arterial blood pressure and central venous pressure monitoring, the pulmonary artery catheter is an essential tool. It is removed by the surgeon during the dissection of the pulmonary arteries and then repositioned. The right heart and pulmonary artery pressures are documented pre-operatively and immediately after the operation, as a decreased MPAP and increase in cardiac output are usually good indicators of operative success. It should be emphasized that the catheter should not be wedged, especially after the endarterectomy as the operated pulmonary vessels may rupture under pressure. A second systemic arterial catheter is routinely inserted in the femoral artery and used to monitor pressure if selective cerebral perfusion is used, and as a guide for the insertion of an intra-aortic balloon pump, if required, to support separation from CPB. It is also important to recognize that there are sometimes substantial differences between systemic blood pressure measured in the radial artery and femoral artery after a long period of CPB or DHCA. Transesophageal echocardiography is a useful tool in assessing right ventricular and left ventricular function, as well as to visualize an ASD, intracardiac thrombi or valvular abnormalities. Temperature monitoring is usually a combination of nasopharyngeal and intravesical temperature monitoring. Electroencephalogram (EEG), somatosensory evoked potential (SSEP) or transcranial near-infrared spectroscopy monitoring have all been advocated as necessary by some to guide the duration of DHCA and assess adequacy of brain perfusion.

INDUCTION

As the right ventricle is hypertrophied in most patients, the main risk on induction is a decrease in perfusion pressure triggering right ventricular ischemia and loss of function. Small dose dopamine and alpha-agonists can be helpful in preventing such an event. Further increases in pulmonary vascular resistance triggered by hypoxia, hypercarbia and decreased cardiac output should be avoided for the same reasons.

MAINTENANCE OF ANESTHESIA

Intravenous anesthesia is preferred to inhalation agents in this patient group due to uncertainty of pulmonary uptake, management during CPB and continued sedation post-operatively.

RESPIRATORY MANAGEMENT

A long-acting muscle relaxant is used to facilitate intubation, and laryngoscopy is conducted only after the administration of large doses of opioids. A single lumen endotracheal tube is sufficient. There is no superior modality of ventilation, but it is recognized that the lung should be ventilated after completion of the dissection with the continuous application of a PEEP of at least 6 cmH_2O (including during transfer from theater to ICU). Failure to do so appears to increase the incidence of reperfusion injury in the immediate post-operative period. Differential ventilation or one-lung ventilation is not required, and of no benefit. Inhaled nitric oxide may be used to improve oxygenation and diminish pulmonary vascular resistance in some patients. However, this intervention does not change outcome.

HEMODYNAMIC SUPPORT

As indicated previously, patients may require a vasoconstrictor on induction to maintain the perfusion pressure and avoid superimposed acute right heart failure. To facilitate separation from CPB, pharmacological support with inotropes and vasopressors may be required. The choice of vasoactive agent will usually depend on institutional preferences, and will be guided by constant use of the TOE. The combination of phosphodiesterase inhibitors such as enoximone and noradrenaline has proven useful in our setting. In our institution, we institute intra-aortic balloon counter-pulsation early on to augment coronary perfusion in the hypertrophied right ventricle.

INTENSIVE CARE MANAGEMENT

Common complications seen after CPB operations (bleeding, arrhythmias and cerebrovascular events) can occur and should be treated appropriately. Post-operative hemorrhage is dealt with according to institutional guidelines, and the transfusion of blood products is usually not required. Specific complications for this procedure are residual pulmonary hypertension and reperfusion injury. Massive pulmonary hemorrhage is also possible and typically happens intra-operatively after completion of the endarterectomy. In the absence of an acute lung injury, respiratory support is gradually reduced over several hours and the patient extubated within the first 24 hours.

RESIDUAL PULMONARY HYPERTENSION

Some patients may have a degree of peripheral disease that has not been recognized pre-operatively while others may not have benefited from a complete surgical clearance. The degree of residual post-operative PVR is a reliable factor to predict mortality but can be improved with iloprost, bosentan or sildenafil. When the operation is successful, MPAP may continue to decrease gradually over several weeks.

REPERFUSION INJURY

Reperfusion injury frequently appears within 48 hours of surgery and is characterized by increased vascular permeability, pulmonary hypertension and leukocyte activation and sequestration in the operated segments. The hypoxemia resulting from it can successfully be treated with inhaled nitric oxide, but, similarly to ARDS, its use has not been shown to improve outcome. Other pharmacological agents such as steroids, prostaglandin E1 and prostacyclin derivatives (intravenously or by inhalation) can also be part of the supportive measures deployed to facilitate lung recovery.

Results

Generally quoted and accepted peri-operative mortality risk is 10%, down to 4% in centers with large experience. In most surviving patients, a marked reduction in the pulmonary arterial pressure is observed and right heart function will return to normal within a few months. Survival at five years is usually greater than 75%.

FURTHER READING

- Dartrevelle P, Fadel E, Mussot S, *et al.* Chronic thromboembolic pulmonary hypertension. *Eur Respir J* 2004; **23**: 637–48.
- Fedullo PF, Auger WR, Kerr KM, Rubin LJ. Chronic thromboembolic pulmonary hypertension. *N Engl J Med* 2001; **345**: 1465–71.
- Manecke GR, Wilson WC, Auger WR, Jamieson SW. Chronic thromboembolic pulmonary hypertension and pulmonary thromboendarterectomy. *Sem Cardiothorac Vasc Anesth* 2005; **9**: 189–204.
- Simon J, Gibbs R, Higenbottam TW. Recommendations on the management of pulmonary hypertension in clinical practice. *Heart* 2001; **86**: i1–i13.

Chapter 16

Anesthesia for esophageal surgery

ABDALLA BANNI

Anatomy

The esophagus is a muscular tube that begins as a continuation of the lower end of the pharynx and ends at the transition into the cardia of the stomach. Topographically, the beginning is at the level of the 6th vertebral body and cricoid cartilage and the end is just below the diaphragm at the level of the 10–12th thoracic vertebra. In the adult the esophagus measures about 25–30 cm, and can be divided into three portions: the cervical, thoracic and abdominal portion. The cervical portion is approximately 5-cm long and lies behind the trachea. The thoracic portion is approximately 20-cm long, begins at the thoracic inlet and extends into the posterior mediastinum. The abdominal portion starts as the esophagus passes through the diaphragmatic hiatus and is approximately 1–3-cm long.

The esophagus has three narrow sections. The uppermost narrowing is 1.5 cm in diameter. It is caused by the cricopharyngeal muscle and functions to close the entrance of the upper esophagus. The middle narrowing is produced by the aortic arch at the tracheal bifurcation. The lowermost diaphragmatic narrowing lies in the esophageal hiatus of the diaphragm and is caused by the gastroesophageal sphincter mechanism.

The esophageal musculature consists of an outer longitudinal and an inner circular layer. The cervical portion contains only striated muscle, whereas in the thoracic and abdominal portion smooth muscle becomes more predominant.

Blood supply to the esophagus is provided by the inferior thyroid artery in the cervical portion, bronchial arteries in combination with direct aortic branches in the thoracic portion, and by the left gastric artery together with the inferior phrenic arteries in the abdominal portion. Due to a T-shaped division of the arteries, the esophagus can be mobilized from the stomach to the level of the aortic arch without causing ischemic necrosis. Venous drainage, via a peri-esophageal venous plexus, parallels arterial supply with the exception that the middle portion drains into the azygos and hemiazygos system. The communication of submucosal venous networks of the esophagus and the stomach allows drainage of portal blood into the superior vena cava in patients with portal hypertension.

The vagal nerve provides parasympathetic innervation of the esophagus. Pain fibers from the esophagus use a combination of sympathetic and parasympathetic pathways, which are also occupied by afferent visceral sensory fibers from the heart, explaining the similar symptomatology of both organs. Both sympathetic and parasympathetic nerves innervate the lower esophageal

Core Topics in Thoracic Anesthesia, ed. Cait P. Searl and Sameena T. Ahmed. Published by Cambridge University Press.

sphincter (LES), but the role of their innervation is unclear.

Indications for surgery

Esophagectomy is commonly performed for cancer of the esophagus and gastric cardia. Barrett's esophagus associated with severe dysplasia, undilatable strictures and benign obstructing tumors may also present for this procedure. In the USA, esophageal cancer occurs in 6:100 000 men and 1.6:100 000 women. It is more common in black people than in white, in males than females, appears most frequently after age 50 and appears to be associated with lower socioeconomic class. From 80–90% of cases are thought to be related to alcohol and cigarette abuse, though other less common toxin exposures have also been incriminated. Squamous cell carcinoma accounts for the majority of esophageal malignancies, but adenocarcinoma is diagnosed with increasing frequency in the cardia or distal esophagus (Barrett's esophagus). The distribution of esophageal carcinoma between the upper, middle and lower thirds of the esophagus is approximately 17–27%, 40–54% and 20–30%, respectively. Unfortunately, it is not the operation but rather the stage and biological behavior of the tumor that determines survival. At the time of diagnosis, only 10% of patients have stage 1 disease and are candidates for curative surgery; 10–25% have stage 2 diseases and are candidates for either curative or palliative surgery; and the remainder have stage 3 disease and the tumor is not resectable for cure.

A multidisciplinary approach and superior surgical outcomes in centers with large caseloads of esophageal resection have supported the case for centralization of patients with esophageal and gastro-esophageal junction (GOJ) cancers. The inverse volume–outcome relationship for esophageal resection has been reported to be one of the strongest. In the UK, centralization of cancer surgery has been recommended since 1995. In 2001 National Health Service (NHS) Executive guidance recommended that cancer centers should expect to operate on at least 100 patients with esophageal cancer and 150 with gastric cancer per year.

Surgical approach

The surgical approach to esophagectomy depends on several factors:

- Anatomic location of tumor.
- Preferred method of reconstruction: transposed stomach, interposed colon, pedicled jejunum.
- Location of the esophageal-enteric anastomosis (cervical vs. thoracic).

The surgical approach (Table 16.1) will determine operative position of the patient, the location of the incision(s), whether or not OLV is indicated, where invasive monitors may be placed, and what type of post-operative pain control is best.

Conventional esophagectomy requires either a laparotomy with a trans-hiatal dissection or laparotomy combined with thoracotomy. Reductions in complication rates have been reported in centers with a high volume of esophageal surgery. As advances in minimally invasive surgical instrumentation and technique continue, some centers have developed the application of minimally invasive techniques to dissect the esophagus in an attempt to further decrease the associated morbidity. At present, most of these case studies or small series use video-assisted thoracoscopy (VATS) to mobilize the thoracic esophagus in combination with a standard open laparotomy to complete the esophagectomy.

Trans-hiatal esophagectomy

A trans-hiatal approach is the most commonly performed operation for esophageal cancer resection. Trans-hiatal esophagectomy is performed in three phases with the patient in a supine position: the abdominal, the mediastinal and the cervical approach. The procedure is initiated through a supraumbilical midline incision extending from the xiphoid to the umbilicus to give access for the distal esophageal dissection. In the following cervical

Table 16.1 Advantages and disadvantages of various surgical approaches.

Surgical approach	Tumor location	Advantages	Disadvantages
Right thoracotomy Via 3rd, 4th, or 5th ICS Midline laparotomy Right or left neck incision	Upper and middle third of the esophagus	Good exposure of the mid-thoracic esophagus. Safer dissection of the Azygos vein in case of infiltration	Need to change patient position. Additional incision increases risk of wound infection
Left thoracotomy 7th or 8th ICS with extension into left abdomen	Middle and lower third of the esophagus	No need to change patient position	Increases the risk of mediastinitis (thoracic location of esophago-enteric anastomosis)
Trans-hiatal esophagectomy (THE) Supraumbilical midline incision Left cervical incision Mediastinal dissection	Upper, middle, or lower third of the esophagus	Decreased mortality compared to transthoracic esophagectomy Decreased pulmonary morbidity Decreased risk of mediastinitis as the esophago-enteric anastomosis is located in the neck	Cardiovascular instability during retrosternal dissection due to compression of heart and great vessels Possible entry into either or both pleural cavities (pneumo-, hemothorax)

phase, the incision parallels the anterior border of the left sternocleidomastoid just below the cricoid cartilage and serves to dissect the proximal esophagus. In the final mediastinal phase, the esophagus is dissected transhiatally by insertion of the surgeon's hand through the abdominal incision. After mobilization of the entire intrathoracic esophagus, division of cervical esophagus, and delivery of the stomach with the attached esophagus out of the abdomen a partial proximal gastrectomy with removal of the esophagus is performed. Finally, after closure of the abdominal incision the cervical esophago-enteric anastomosis is performed and the cervical wound is closed.

Trans-hiatal esophagectomy is only a palliative procedure for intrathoracic esophageal cancer because it does not include resection of mediastinal lymph nodes or other potentially resectable structures. This approach is used for a curative resection of tumors of the lower third of the esophagus or gastric cardia.

Pre-anesthetic and pre-operative evaluation

Patients with potentially resectable tumor and curative surgery should not be denied their chance. However, a balance has to be reached between what is surgically possible and the patient's chances of surviving the procedure. Usually the anesthetists are only involved in the patient's management further along the line after the decisions about surgery have been made. This gives the anesthetists little

Table 16.2 Organ-system pre-anesthetic evaluation.

System	Effect	History	Physical exam	Test
Cardiac	Coronary artery diease-left ventricle dysfunction, pulmonary hypertension, right ventricle dysfunction, dilated cardiomyopathy	Angina dyspnea, orthopnea, paroxysmal nocturnal dyspnea palpitations	Heart sounds S3, S4, fixed split S2 displaced point of maximum (cardiac) impulse, irregular rhythm	ECG, ECHO, stress test and cardiopulmonary exercise tests
Pulmonary	COPD (tobacco abuse) Restrictive lung disease (chronic aspiration) Pulmonary fibrosis (bleomycin) Pneumonitis (radiation therapy)	Shortness of breath/exercise tolerance, cough, sputum production recurrent pneumonias	Prolonged I:E, wheezing	Chest X-ray, PFTs
CNS	Delirium tremens	ETOH consumption		
Gastro-intestinal	Dysphagia and liver cirrhosis	Limited oral intake, heart burn, regurgitation	Dehydration, orthostatic jaundice	Liver function tests
Genito-urinary	Renal insufficiency		Urine production	BUN/Creatinine and electrolytes
Hematology	Anemia	Fatigue	Pallor	Complete blood count
General	Weakness	Poor nutrition	Muscle wasting	Albumin

chance to be fully involved in the decision-making process as peri-operative physicians. The patients usually present with dysphagia and weight loss. Sadly, the disease has already spread by this stage. The lack of serosal layer around the esophagus and the presense of an extensive lymphatic system results in spread of the tumor to the liver and the lungs. Risk factors that can increase peri-operative mortality include impairment of cardiac function, hepatic function due to chronic alcohol use and respiratory function from tobacco usage (Table 16.2).

The patient's general condition must be optimized. This will require pre-operative correction of anemia, dehydration and electrolyte imbalance. Pre-operative parenteral nutrition should be considered if the patient is severely malnourished and an oral diet has been unsuccessful, since this improves the outcome. Acute chest infection sec-ondary to aspiration of the esophageal contents should be treated with antibiotics and chest physio-therapy. Evidence of chronic pulmonary disease, the ability to stand one-lung anesthesia and the like-lihood of post-operative pulmonary complications may be predicted with the aid of the lung function test and cardiopulmonary exercise testing.

There is growing opinion that neo-adjuvant chemotherapy (NAC) is effective in improving survival. The potential benefits of NAC administration include improvement of swallowing, resulting in better patient nutrition, down-staging of the primary tumor and elimination of micro-metastases, thus increasing the likelihood of a curative resection. In the UK, current guidelines suggest that pre-operative chemotherapy for adenocarcinoma and squamous cell carcinoma of the esophagus and esophago-gastric junction (OGJ) (types I and

Table 16.3 Invasive monitoring during esophagectomy.

Monitoring	Indications	Comments
A-LINE	BP (LV/RV dysfunction, manipulation of heart), arterial blood gases (chronic lung disease, OLV, esophageal-pulmonary fistula)	Place pre-operatively given the possibility of a hypovolemic state
CVP	Pre load assessment Central administration of drugs	3-lumen if good peripheral access otherwise 9 Fr introducer sheath
PA catheter	Pre-load assessment: consider in pts. with LV or RV dysfunction, and pulmonary hypertension	No conclusive data to support use

II) should be considered. Patients present for surgery within 5–6 weeks of NAC. This can have implications for the anesthetists. Adequate vascular access is required for effective administration of chemotherapeutic agents, blood products, nutritional support and the multiple blood tests needed for monitoring cancer patients. This can present the anesthetist with difficult peripheral venous access at induction. Neutropenia can occur either due to the malignant process or chemotherapy-induced bone marrow myelosuppression. Neutropenic patients are at increased risk of developing opportunistic infection. Infection in hospitalized oncology patients poses a serious challenge with unfavorable outcome. Myelosuppression with thrombocytopenia poses a problem for insertion of thoracic epidurals.

All patients undergoing esophagectomy should have the following investigations performed pre-operatively:

- Full blood count.
- Urea creatinine and electrolytes.
- Liver function test.
- Blood glucose.
- Blood grouping and cross matching.
- Sputum culture and sensitivity.
- Lung function test.
- Chest radiograph.
- Electrocardiogram.

In addition, patients who present for esophageal resection are further evaluated with bone scan, upper gastrointestinal studies, CT of chest and abdomen and endoscopies with biopsies.

Anesthetic room set-up

- 2 IV setup with blood tubing and pressure bags.
- 1–2 blood-warmers, Bair Hugger (lower body).
- Arterial-line and CVP or pulmonary arterial catheter set-up (if indicated – see below).
- Double-lumen tube vs. Univent vs. regular endotracheal tube with Arndt bronchial blocker if thoracotomy is planned.
- Fiberoptic bronchoscope.
- A bean bag in place on the table if lateral decubitus position is planned.
- Keep room temperature up until patient is prepped and draped.

Monitoring

Be sure placement and dressing of the central line will not interfere with any planned cervical incision. Check with surgeon which side of the neck to use for venous access (Table 16.3).

Pre-operative considerations

- Continue cardiac and antihypertensive medication (especially beta-blockers) up to time of surgery.
- Prophylactic anti-aspiration regimen.
- Careful sedation not to obtund a patient at risk for aspiration.
- Antibiotic prophylaxis. According to guidelines written by the Section of Thoracic Surgery, all

Table 16.4 Considerations for patient positioning during surgery.

Lateral decubitus position (thoracotomy)	Supine position (trans-hiatal esophagectomy)
• Bean bag and head rest (foam donut or pillow)	• Headrest with neck exposure for cervical anastomosis
• Maintain perfusion to the down arm and prevent stretching of the suprascapular nerve	• Arms tucked and padded
• Support dependent arm on arm board	
• Position the hips at break in table	
• Ascertain that the genitalia in males are not strangulated	
• Support lower extremities to prevent compression necrosis of skin overlying bony structures	
• A strap (or tape) between the iliac crest and the femoral head to stabilize the lower torso	

esophageal resections will receive prophylactic antibiotics. The first dose should be given prior to incision, in the pre-op holding area. Generally, a broad spectrum cephalosporin is used, unless the colon is to be opened. Antibiotics are continued for the first 24 hours.

• Patients should be cross-matched for four units of blood at least.

• There are no specific requirements for pre-medication. Neutralization of the gastric PH is not specifically indicated. Drainage of the fluid esophageal content proximal to the obstruction can be performed with a naso-gastric tube.

Induction of anesthesia and airway management

All patients with carcinoma of the esophagus are at risk from regurgitation and aspiration of the esophago-gastric contents. Gastro-esophageal reflux is a risk factor for the development of esophageal cancer. Food can collect proximal to an esophageal obstruction. This may not clear after an overnight fast. Most patients undergoing esophageal surgery are thus at risk of aspiration at induction. Rapid sequence induction with cricoid

pressure in a head-up tilt position is recommended in all cases unless contraindicated. Patients with hypoalbuminemia will have a rapid increase in the concentration of the free induction agent and rapid injecting can cause profound hemodynamic changes.

A double lumen endotracheal tube is usually inserted if a thoracotomy approach is used. This will allow easier access to the esophagus with a collapse of uppermost lung. A left-side tube is safer to use.

• Rapid sequence intubation with cricoid pressure and head-up tilt (consider orogastric/ neurogastric aspiration of pouch above stricture).

• Awake FOB intubation in patient with difficult airway.

• Monitor blood pressure closely in light of possibility of hypovolemia.

Intra-operative considerations: positioning

Depending on the surgical approach, the patient may remain supine throughout the procedure, in lateral decubitus for a thoracotomy throughout the surgery, or moved from supine to lateral or vice versa (Table 16.4).

Various anesthetic techniques are used as no single technique has been shown to be superior. These include:

1. GA with single shot spinal opiates or post-op patient-controlled analgesia.
2. Combined GA/EA with post-op thoracic EA.
3. GA with post-op thoracic EA.

Continuous thoracic epidurals are accepted as state-of-the-art for post-thoracotomy pain control. Avoid N_2O in the setting of one-lung ventilation or if a colonic interposition is planned. Closely monitor blood loss and maintain intravascular volume and blood loss. The anesthetist should be aware of the possibility of severe hypotension and dysrhythmias from mediastinal compression (particularly during a trans-hiatal approach). This requires close communication with the surgeon. Other problems during surgery include dislodgement of the endotracheal tube, perforation of the mediastinal pleura resulting in pneumo- or hemothorax and injury to the posterior membranous wall of the trachea.

During cervical anastomosis, an over-sized endotracheal tube cuff may interfere by pushing the posterior tracheal membrane into the anterior surface of the esophagus.

Post-operative care

The main objective of the post-operative period is to ensure a rapid weaning from respiratory support with stability of the respiratory and cardiovascular functions, warranting good anastomosis healing. Some clinicians emphasize routine early extubation, while others prefer elective overnight ventilation. Early extubation has been advocated to reduce morbidity and cost after esophagectomy. Current literature supports early extubation as safe and associated with reduced intensive care stay. Patients can be extubated if they are hemodynamically stable, warm and alert with no residual muscle relaxation and adequate analgesia.

Risk factors for gastric content aspiration after esophagectomy are:

- Creation of an esophago-gastric anastomosis.
- Recurrent laryngeal nerve injury.
- Vagus nerve damage resulting in dysfunction of the cricopharyngeal sphincter muscle.

Problems that may complicate esophagectomy and affect the post-operative anesthetic care include:

- Poor analgesia with splinting, particularly after thoracotomy – a multimodal approach consisting of PCA or epidural analgesia, aggressive physiotherapy and early mobilization is the key!
- Pulmonary complications, particularly with thoracotomy, are the leading cause of peri-operative morbidity (atelectasis, pulmonary edema, pneumo-, hemo-, chylothorax, pleural effusion and aspiration syndrome).
- Mediastinitis due to a leak of a thoracic esophageal enteric anastomosis.
- CLN injury due to a leak of a cervical esophageal enteric anastomosis.
- Delayed gastric emptying – depends on drainage procedure.
- Herniation of abdominal viscera through diaphragm – rare.

The recent Confidential Enquiry into Peri-Operative Deaths (CEPOP) recorded "respiratory problems as being a major cause of morbidity and mortality after elective oesophageal surgery." This conclusion is supported by many published reports and a systematic review. The incidence of respiratory problems after esophagectomy is about 27%. This could be due to multiple factors:

- Long periods of one-lung ventilation (OLV).
- Aspiration of gastric contents.
- Poor pain control after surgery. Thoracic epidurals not producing the desired pain control should be re-sited earlier.
- Mechanical ventilation with relatively high tidal volumes used during OLV could result in ventilator-induced lung injury.

- Peri-operative endotoxemia and release of proinflammatory cytokines.

Factors associated with increased mortality include increasing age, poor nutritional state, poor lung function, borderline arterial blood gases and the presence of chronic respiratory and liver disease.

Anesthetic management for gastro-esophageal reflux surgery

The spectrum of gastro-esophageal reflux disease (GERD) involves the gastrointestinal and pulmonary organ systems. The American College of Gastroenterology defines GERD as "chronic symptoms or mucosal damage produced by the abnormal reflux of gastric contents into the esophagus." The symptoms of GERD and the symptoms of pulmonary diseases have been recognized since the beginning of time.

Currently, the number of individuals with GERD symptoms in the USA alone is estimated to be in the range of 30 million and in Asia, with its vastly larger population, up to 3- or 4-fold more. Although the disease was initially considered to be predominantly a problem of Western society, it is now apparent that the East is currently experiencing a considerable increase in GERD, and it seems that the development of the disease in Asia will, within a decade, mirror what has taken place in the West. For the majority of patients, this is a self-limited condition that may be improved with changes in lifestyle or medical therapy. However, approximately 25% of patients with GERD will develop progressive disease that does not respond to simple therapy and may benefit from an anti-reflux procedure. There is an association between GERD and end-stage lung disease, especially idiopathic pulmonary fibrosis (IPF). The presence of GERD may predispose to the development of bronchiolitis obliterans following lung transplantation. It is presently unclear what effect surgical correction of GERD may have in the progression of underlying native lung disease. Nissan's fundoplication can be carried out safely in patients with documented GERD awaiting lung transplantation.

Clinical presentation

Small-sized hernias are usually asymptomatic. The patient gives a long history of post-prandial distress or discomfort with substernal fullness and belching. Sometimes dysphagia can occur. Pulmonary complications are common: recurrent pneumonia; chronic atelectasis; dyspnea especially after a large meal from pleural space compression by the huge hernial sac.

The patient can develop ulceration of the herniated stomach with resultant bleeding and anemia. Obese patients with hiatus hernia can have impaired respiratory functions due to both obesity and the presence of abdominal structures in the thorax. These patients should have pulmonary function tests.

A chest X-ray will show retro-cardiac air-fluid level and a barium swallow will show an intrathoracic stomach.

Surgical considerations

Hiatus hernia is present in a large number of patients with GERD. Two types of hiatus hernia can occur.

- Type 1 or sliding hernia. This constitutes the majority of cases. The gastro-esophageal junction and fundus of the stomach herniate through the esophageal hiatus into the thorax.
- Type 2 or para-esophageal hernia. A portion of the stomach herniates through the hiatus next to the esophagus. The gastro-esophageal junction remains within the abdomen.

The aim of surgery is to increase the gastro-esophageal junction competency. Various surgical techniques have been developed, the commonest being Nissen's fundoplication. This is performed laparoscopically which allows faster recovery and lesser post-operative pain. During the procedure, there is a risk of esophageal perforation from passing the esophageal boogie dilator. This requires converting the laparoscopy to an open procedure. Depending upon the position of the tear, a thoracotomy may be required. Laparoscopic Nissen fundoplication is a well-proven therapy for gastro-esophageal reflux disease, with over 90% of patients being highly satisfied on 8–10 year follow-up.

Anesthetic considerations

Patients with an incomplete lower esophageal sphincter are at risk of reflux and aspiration of gastric contents. They should all receive pre-operative H_2 blockers or proton pump inhibitors. Omeprazole 20 mg given pre-operatively has been shown to reduce both acidity and volume of gastric fluids. Metaclopromide 10 mg intravenously can increase lower esophageal sphincter tone. A rapid sequence induction technique with cricoid pressure should be used with the patient in a semi-recumbent position. A single lumen tube can be used to secure the airway.

The patient is placed in a modified lithotomy position with the head of the table tilted up 25 degrees. The operating surgeon stands between the patient's legs while the camera operator stands to the patient's right and the second assistant assumes a position on the patient's left.

Post-operative recovery

Patients are allowed to take liquids on recovery from anesthesia and are maintained on a diet of pureed foods for 1–2 weeks. Analgesia is given in liquid form for the first 2 weeks and all pills are crushed. Most patients are allowed to leave hospital on the first post-operative day.

FURTHER READING

- Al-Sarira AA, David G, Willmott S, *et al.* Oesophagectomy practice and outcomes in England. *Br J Surg* 2007; **94(5)**: 585–91.
- Benumof J. Anesthesia for esophageal surgery. In Benumof J, ed. *Anesthesia for Thoracic Surgery*, 2nd edn. Saunders, 1995.
- Dupont FW. Anesthesia for esophageal surgery. *Sem Cardiothorac Vasc Anesth* 2000; 4: 2–17.
- Kavanagh BP, Katz J, Sandler AN. Pain control after thoracic surgery. A review of current techniques. *Anesthesiology* 1994; **81**: 737–59.
- Oberhelman HA, Howard SK. Oesophagectomy. In Jaffe RA, Samuel SI, eds. *Anesthesiologists Manual of Surgical Procedures*, 2nd edn. Raven Press, 1999.
- Sugarbaker DJ, DeCamp MM. Selecting the surgical approach to cancer of the esophagus. *Chest* 1993; **103**: 410S–14S.
- Sontag SJ. The spectrum of gastroesophageal reflux disease. *J Clin Gastroenterol* 2007; **41** (Suppl. 2): 118S–28S.

Chapter 17

Anesthesia for pleural and chest wall surgery

CAIT P. SEARL

In addition to allowing therapeutic surgery to the lungs, the use of one-lung anesthesia is utilized in the management of other thoracic disorders including those of the pleura and chest wall. These procedures represent a heterogenous group and the underlying pathology can often represent the main challenge to the anesthetist rather than the surgical requirements.

Procedures on the pleura
Pleurectomy

Pleurectomy is the removal of the parietal layer of pleura from the chest wall and is generally performed to prevent recurrence of pneumothorax. This may be performed as an open thoracotomy but is generally performed as a video-assisted thoracoscopic procedure. Patients presenting for pleurectomy often have associated lung diseases such as asthma, emphysema and cystic fibrosis. Appropriate pre-operative optimizing of their condition should occur. The patient may have a chest drain in situ for an established pneumothorax (Figure 17.1). This should be left unclamped during the induction of anesthesia and during subsequent ventilation to prevent development of a tension pneumothorax. The use of nitrous oxide is usually avoided. One-lung anesthesia is required to assist access for this procedure during which the pleura is stripped

where possible. Mechanical abrasion is performed to deliberately cause inflammation and promote adhesion formation. A chest drain is positioned at the end of the procedure to assist expansion of the lung and to allow drainage of blood. This operation can cause extreme pain and analgesia needs to reflect this. Thoracic epidural or paravertebral block should be considered. The patient should be initially cared for in a high-dependency unit to allow optimization of analgesia and management of the chest drain.

Pleurodesis

Pleurodesis is the use of talc or other irritant to produce inflammation of the visceral and parietal pleural surfaces with resultant obliteration of the pleural space. It may be performed to treat recurrent pneumothorax, particularly in patients who are unfit for the more invasive pleurectomy and in patients in whom lung transplantation may be a future option (e.g. with cystic fibrosis or lymphangioleiomyomatosis). Pleurodesis is also employed in the prevention of pleural effusions, particularly in malignant disease. The procedure is usually performed thoracoscopically and is short in duration. One-lung anesthesia is not always necessary but may assist and therefore further shorten the procedure. Pleurodesis causes a considerable amount

Core Topics in Thoracic Anesthesia, ed. Cait P. Searl and Sameena T. Ahmed. Published by Cambridge University Press.
© Cambridge University Press 2009.

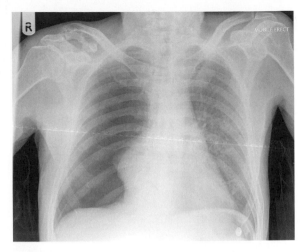

Figure 17.1 A right-sided pneumothorax on chest X-ray.

> **Box 17.1** Principles of treatment of empyema
>
> General supportive measures.
> Antimicrobial therapy: ideally based on the results of blood and pleural fluid microbiological cultures and sensitivities.
> Drainage: Drainage of pleural effusions is indicated when the effusion is turbid or purulent or loculated. It is also indicated if micro-organisms are identified in the pleural fluid or if the fluid has a pH below 7.2 in association with a pneumonic illness. In the first instance this may be done non-surgically.
> Surgical management: Surgical interventions for the management of empyema include VATS debridement; thoracotomy with decortication; and open thoracic drainage. There are no published randomized trials to guide surgical intervention.

of post-operative pain as the point of the procedure is to induce inflammation. Again it is important to optimize analgesia to ensure adequate post-operative respiratory function. A chest drain is usually placed until fluid, including blood, and air stop draining.

Surgical management of empyema

An empyema is a collection of pus in the pleural space. It is a dangerous condition developing most often as a complication of pneumonia. It can be complicated by the development of septicemia and disseminated abscess formation and mortality can exceed 50% in elderly patients or patients with significant comorbidities. Although the commonest association of bacterial infection of the pleural space is a concomitant pneumonia, other causes include trauma or surgery to the thorax; extension of a suppurative process from either neck or abdomen; and hematogenous spread of infection from elsewhere in the body.

The indications for primary surgical intervention are not clearly defined but usually include failure of non-surgical management and the persistence of septic features. These patients are often at the sicker end of the spectrum of patients with empyema and can be challenging anesthetically due to the associated morbidity of long-term sepsis (Box 17.1). Over half of patients presenting with empyema have concomitant chronic disease (e.g. diabetes mellitus; malignancy) or conditions that predispose to aspiration pneumonia (e.g. alcohol abuse).

Thoracoscopy and VAT debridement: Under general anesthetic and with one-lung ventilation, a thoracoscope is inserted into the pleural space, visually enabling the use of forceps to break down adhesions and a suction catheter for drainage. VATS is frequently unsuccessful in empyema owing to the thickening of the pleura. The thickened cortex on the visceral pleura prevents the re-expansion of the underlying lung. The anesthetist therefore must be prepared for the likelihood of conversion to thoracotomy and decortication.

Thoracotomy and decortication: Decortication is a major surgical procedure involving the removal of the cortex on the visceral pleura. It is more likely to be necessary in patients with multiloculated empyema; illness of greater than 4 weeks; or if there is > 25% impairment of lung expansion. Decortication is often associated with significant

Box 17.2 Congenital chest wall deformities

Pectus excavatum (funnel chest).
Pectus carinatum (pigeon chest).
Cleft sternum.
Poland syndrome (congenital absence of breast, associated pectus muscle and underlying ribs).

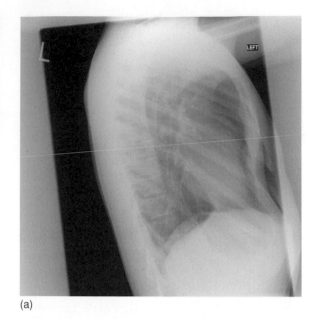

(a)

peri-operative blood loss, due in part to the severity of adhesions and to the continuing inflammation.

Open drainage: In patients whose frailty precludes a major thoracotomy procedure, it is possible to do a rib resection with manual breakdown of adhesions/loculations and drainage of the pleural space. This can be achieved under local anesthesia with sedation where general anesthesia is felt to be too risky to proceed with. This results in an open chest wound for around 6 months.

Chest wall procedures

These are divisible into those performed to treat congenital chest wall disorders and those for acquired disease. Congenital deformities can arise from abnormal development of the sternum, costal cartilages and/or ribs (Box 17.2). The commonest congenital deformity presenting for surgery is pectus excavatum. This has varying degrees of severity and is associated with a spectrum of symptoms from psychological distress to shortness of breath. At the severe end of the spectrum, pectus excavatum is associated with cardiac dysfunction secondary to sternal compression of the right ventricle (Figure 17.2). This does not necessarily resolve with the correction of the deformity. Pectus excavatum is also associated with other musculoskeletal disorders such as scoliosis and with connective tissue disorders such as Marfan's syndrome. A variety of surgical solutions are employed (see Box 17.3). Careful pre-assessment of these patients is required, as although mainly young and 'fit' the presence of other problems may only become apparent on careful questioning and examination.

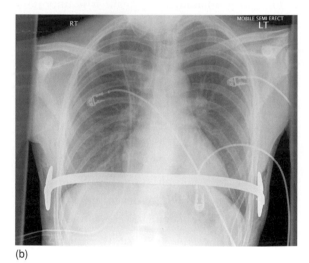

(b)

Figure 17.2. (a) A lateral chest X-ray showing pectus excavatum (funnel chest); (b) PA chest X-ray following a Nuss procedure.

Lung function tests may be helpful in assessment of potential restrictive lung function and a transthoracic echo may reassure as to cardiac function. A lateral chest X-ray may establish proximity of the sternum to cardiac structures. All the surgical procedures can cause considerable analgesic requirements post-operatively.

Box 17.3 Surgical procedures for correction of pectus excavatum

"Turnover" technique: still employed with some severe deformities, the sternal bone is essentially resected and replaced inverted; associated with a high rate of sternal necrosis due to disruption of the blood supply.

Ravitch procedure: consists of resection of abnormal cartilages, followed by a transverse anterior sternal osteotomy to allow anterior displacement of the sternum and then sternal fixation to prevent posterior displacement.

Nuss procedure: this is a "minimally invasive" procedure with the placement of a bar to displace the sternum forwards; this is usually left in place around 2 years; this is supported by good results reported in a large case series.

The commonest set of operations for acquired chest wall disorders are those requiring chest wall resection. This may be for the treatment of "benign" disease such as osteomyelitis or for malignant neoplasms, primary or secondary. Chest wall resection requires careful operative planning including the extent of resection, the options for chest wall stabilization and the method of tissue coverage to be employed, usually a muscle flap. Such procedures are often multidisciplinary, requiring cooperation between specialists beyond thoracic surgery, including in plastic surgery. It is the author's experience that these procedures can be extremely long in duration and require careful positioning of the patient to prevent pressure problems. Although warming devices are used, maintenance of normal body temperature may be difficult to achieve with exposure of large areas of the thorax. Invasive monitoring is useful and good venous access essential. In our center these patients are usually admitted to intensive care post-operatively and a period of post-operative invasive ventilation may be considered especially where analgesia may be difficult to establish to satisfactory levels and to allow correction to normal body temperature. Special attention should be paid to post-operative analgesia. Patients who have undergone extensive resection often will already also have longstanding pain issues and may already be on considerable amounts of sustained release morphine and other analgesics. We employ regional techniques, particularly epidurals, to supplement other analgesic modalities. Pain is likely to compound post-operative atelectasis and pneumonia can result from sputum retention.

Chapter 18

Anesthetic implications for management of thoracic trauma

SAMEENA T. AHMED

Thoracic trauma accounts for 25% of all trauma-related deaths. Significant thoracic trauma is present in more than 50% of fatal road crashes. Injuries can occur to the chest wall, lungs and pleura, thoracic great vessels, diaphragm, heart, trachea, bronchus and esophagus. The magnitude and significance of these injuries is important for the complete evaluation and management of thoracic trauma patients. As the care of patients with thoracic trauma calls for particular attention to the management of airway, ventilation and hemodynamic status, an anesthetist is a vital member of the multidisciplinary team. Only 10–15% of blunt trauma and 15–30% of penetrating chest trauma requires thoracic surgery. The majority of thoracic trauma patients can be managed conservatively by simple chest tube drainage, respiratory support and pain management.

Secondary injuries from thoracic trauma also have significant morbidity and mortality. Pneumonia, acute lung injury or acute respiratory distress syndromes (ARDS) are clearly associated with long stays in intensive care. Over the last 15 years, faster and more detailed diagnosis of thoracic injuries has been achieved by computerized tomography. Morbidity and mortality of thoracic trauma have been reduced by new surgical techniques such as video-assisted thoracoscopic surgery (VATS) and devel-

opments in extracorporeal membrane oxygenation (ECMO) and endovascular stenting of thoracic aortic disruption. All these techniques have made their contributions to a growing complexity of acute and intensive care of thoracic trauma.

Application of the fundamental principles of initial trauma management can substantially reduce the morbidity and mortality. Appropriate early management of the rapidly progressing and potentially fatal thoracic injuries can also significantly decrease the late complications. Optimal treatment requires a thorough knowledge of the etiology of the injury mechanisms and pathology inflicted by them on the thoracic organs. Improved pre-hospital care and rapid transportation have increased the survival, but the mortality remains high.

Mechanism of injury after thoracic trauma

The mechanism of injury can be classified as blunt or penetrating trauma. In addition, blast injury has a specific action on the thoracic organs. This injury usually occurs during military conflicts. However, recent bombings around the world have emphasized that no community is completely safe from deliberate explosions.

> **Box 18.1** Factors that determine the severity of gunshot wounds
>
> 1. Mass and velocity of the bullet.
> 2. Kinetic energy of the bullet.
> 3. Shape and stability of the bullet.
> 4. Tissue density. Greater damage seen when denser tissue is struck. There is more retardation of the bullet allowing for more transfer of energy.
> 5. Cavitations and shock waves. High energy bullets set up temporary cavitations and shock waves causing tissue destruction.

Penetrating wounds

These occur due to gunshots and stabbings. Gun shots are destructive due to the kinetic energy transmitted to the body on impact. This sets up a pressure wave which can destroy a wide area of tissues and organs. The amount of destruction caused by gunshot wounds can be calculated from the amount of kinetic energy transmitted to the tissues.

Kinetic energy $= WV^2/2G$. (W = weight; V = velocity; G = acceleration of gravity.)

Rifle bullets in the past depended upon their mass and shape to produce injury. Modern guns have considerably reduced bullets and very high velocity. The severity of injury caused by gunshot wounds has increased considerably (Box 18.1).

Stabbing wounds are less complex. The tissue damage is limited to the structures in the path of the knife. In most cases of stabbing, the knife is found to be in place at the time medical personnel arrive at the scene. Embedded foreign bodies are present more often in accidental penetrating chest injuries. Extraction of embedded objects from the chest can result in major bleeding, hemodynamic deterioration and rapid death of the victim. They should be removed under direct vision in the operating room. Sternotomy, thoracotomy and the VATS approach have been used to extract embedded knives from the chest. Most patients with penetrating cardiac injuries die at the scene of accident. Rapid surgical intervention can lead to a successful outcome. Stab wounds have a mortality of 15.6% if treated surgically. In contrast, the mortality is 81% in patients with gunshot wounds of the heart.

Blunt injuries

The majority of blunt trauma to the chest is due to road traffic accidents. The mechanism of injury can be due to:

1. Rapid deceleration.
2. Direct impact.
3. Compression.

Rapid deceleration occurs in road traffic accidents and in falls from a height. Deceleration force can cause injuries from momentum and impact. Momentum is the force that carried the person forward by virtue of mass and velocity. Momentum injuries occur to the organs that are suspended within the chest cavity such as the lungs, heart and vascular structures (aorta, innominate artery, pulmonary veins and vena cavae). Rupture of the descending aorta at the isthmus is a common feature of severe deceleration injury. The degree of external trauma and bruising may not fully predict the severity of internal injuries. Direct impact injuries can cause fractures of the ribs, sternum or scapula with underlying lung parenchyma injury, cardiac contusion and pneumothorax.

Compression of the chest prevents respiration and causes marked increases in venous pressure. It can result in traumatic asphyxia. Anterior-posterior compression forces cause lateral and mid-shaft rib fractures. Lateral compression forces cause sterno-clavicular joint dislocation and clavicle fractures.

Blast injuries

An explosion is defined as the release of mechanical, chemical or nuclear energy in a sudden and often violent manner with generation of high temperatures and winds. The abrupt rise in atmospheric

Box 18.2 Mechanism of blast injury to the thoracic structures

Organ system	Effects
The larynx and trachea	Thermal injury, hemorrhages on the vocal cords, dislocation of cartilages, or laryngeal fracture. These can make intubation difficult. Bronchoscopy recommended to determine the extent of injury to the major airways.
The lungs	It is characterized by apnea, bradycardia and hypotension. Primary blast and flying shrapnel can cause pneumothorax, hemothorax, pneumo-mediastinum, subcutaneous emphysema and pulmonary contusion. The blast overpressure can cause disruption of the alveolar-capillary interface leading to life-threatening air embolism.
The heart	Cardiac contusion and myocardial ischemia caused by air or other emboli are major causes of death. Cardiac arrhythmias including asystole and ventricular fibrillation are common. Blast-induced shock may result from immediate myocardial depression without a compensatory vasoconstriction.

pressure is termed "blast overpressure." The leading front of this pressure wave, termed "blast front" is responsible for the peak high pressure. If the pressure wave is reflected by a solid surface, the reflected pressure increases several times that of the incident wave. Injury and mortality can therefore be much higher if the victim is in close proximity to solid structures. The same principle is valid for confined space explosions. Life-threatening multi-organ injuries may occur to many victims simultaneously. Injuries mostly occur to the hollow organs, in particular the lungs, gastrointestinal tract and the ears. Development of air emboli in the pulmonary and systemic circulations are the main mechanisms leading to death from the blast itself. The clinical picture could change over time and patients who had been self-ventilating can end up requiring endotracheal intubation (Box 18.2).

Anesthetic implications for management of thoracic trauma

The majority of patients with thoracic trauma can be managed conservatively. However, a small but significant number require emergency thoracotomy or sternotomy as part of their initial resuscitation. The anesthetist plays an important role in the management of severe thoracic trauma from an initial stage of primary survey right through to management in the intensive care unit. Pneumonia, acute lung injury and acute respiratory distress syndrome (ARDS) are associated with long stays in intensive care.

Emergency management

In the emergency department, decisions and actions have to be taken without delay. In a trauma situation, there is little opportunity to obtain standard anesthetic pre-operative assessment. Important information can be obtained from the ambulance services about the patient's relevant history, the mechanism of injury, treatment given at the site and vital signs of the patient. Respiratory rate is an important part of this but often overlooked.

The patient should be resuscitated based upon well-described trauma guidelines. The approach can be divided into four main components:
1. Primary survey.
2. Resuscitation of vital function.
3. Secondary survey.
4. Definitive care.

The initial priorities of managing all trauma patients are airway and breathing management with cervical spine immobilization, evaluating and establishing circulation and assessing level of consciousness.

Box 18.3 The "Deadly Dozen" major thoracic injuries

Lethal injuries which should be diagnosed and treated during the primary survey	Hidden injuries which should be diagnosed during the secondary survey
Airway obstruction. Tension pneumothorax.	Myocardial contusion. Tracheo-bronchial disruption.
Cardiac tamponade.	Disruption of the thoracic aorta.
Open pneumothorax. Massive hemothorax. Flail chest.	Diaphragmatic tear. Esophageal tear. Lung contusion.

The primary survey with simultaneous resuscitation is carried out until the patient is stable. The secondary survey and investigations are only performed on a stable trauma patient. The main consequences of chest trauma are respiratory and hemodynamic disruption. This manifests as hypoxia and hypoperfusion.

Major thoracic injuries are known as the "deadly dozen": these are the "Lethal six" and the "Hidden six" (Box 18.3).

Assessment of patients with thoracic trauma

The chest must be fully exposed to assess the respiratory rate and mechanism of breathing (Table 18.1). Inspection and palpation of the chest wall can show deformity, contusions, penetrating injury, tenderness, instability or subcutaneous emphysema. Auscultation of the chest is performed to assess air entry on each side. Absence of air entry on one side is an indication of massive hemothorax or tension pneumothorax. A formal assessment of the back of the chest can be done as part of the log roll. This must be done earlier in patients with penetrating trauma to detect life-threatening wounds.

Bruising and wounds over the chest will highlight the likelihood of underlying injury. However, most thoracic injuries can occur without any external damage. In a road traffic accident, bruising from a seat belt is suspicious of rib fractures and lung contusion. Steering wheel injury is suspicious of myocardial contusion and cardiac tamponade. Any penetrating injury medial to the nipples or scapula indicates trauma to the heart and hilar structures. Venous distension of the neck veins may not be present in patients with cardiac tamponade if they are hypovolemic. Fractures of the first or second ribs should alert the doctor to be suspicious of aortic disruption.

Fluid management in patients with thoracic trauma

Venous access should be established as early as possible. Two large bore venous cannulae should be inserted. Facilities for central venous catheters and venous cut-down should be available. A urinary catheter should be inserted as soon as possible. Fluid replacement is a key to successful resuscitation after major trauma. The traditional approach for managing patients presenting with low blood pressure, presumably from hemorrhage, has been to correct the blood pressure.

Bickell *et al.* in 1994 conducted a prospective controlled clinical trial comparing immediate pre-operative intravenous fluid resuscitation with delayed fluid resuscitation until arrival in the operating room in Houston, USA. They found that patients in the pre-operative resuscitation group had a higher mortality rate and a higher rate of post-operative complications compared with patients in the delayed resuscitation group. They concluded that elevation of blood pressure is beneficial only after hemorrhage is controlled. The potential mechanisms for the worse outcome could be:

- Acceleration of ongoing hemorrhage as a result of the elevated blood pressure.
- Dissolution of soft clot formation.

Table 18.1 Outlining presentation and treatment of life-threatening thoracic injuries.

Open pneumothorax	**Treatment**
This is a penetrating wound of the chest creating a communication between the pleural space and external environment	Initially apply a sterile occlusive dressing large enough to cover the wound and taped securely on three sides
Defects larger than two thirds the size of the tracheal diameter cause air to preferentially pass through the lower resistance injury tract rather than through the normal airways	A chest tube drain should be inserted at a remote site
It produces a "sucking" wound on the chest wall	In small chest wall defects, the pleura may soon seal and no further intervention is necessary. Often surgical repair is required
Tension pneumothorax	**Treatment**
Air enters the pleural cavity through a lung wound or penetrating chest wound with valve-like opening	Immediate chest tube insertion with underwater-seal drainage
Ipsilateral lung collapses and mediastinum shifts to opposite side compressing contralateral lung	If the lung does not fully re-expand or there is a large ongoing air leak the airways should be evaluated with a bronchoscope to exclude major tracheo-bronchial injury
Progressively increasing intrathoracic pressure in the affected side results in impaired central venous return and mediastinal shift	
Chest X-ray demonstrates trachea and mediastinum deviation to the opposite side of the tension pneumothorax, while on the ipsilateral side intercostal spaces are widened and the diaphragm is pushed downward	
Massive hemothorax	**Treatment**
Hemodynamic instability develops due to loss of intravascular volume and compromised central venous return	Large chest tube insertion
Lung compression from massive blood accumulation causes respiratory compromise	A hemothorax > 1500–2000 ml or continuous bleeding of > 250 ml/hour is an indication for emergency thoracotomy or VAT
The diagnosis is readily made from the clinical picture and X-ray evidence of fluid in the pleural space	Massive clots may lead to respiratory difficulty and infection, and should be evacuated surgically. Small clots will re-absorbed
Cardiac tamponade	**Treatment**
There should be a high degree of suspicion of cardiac injury in chest trauma	Prompt definitive therapy is imperative
The immediate cause of death is exsanguination, cardiac tamponade or interference with the conduction mechanism	This includes emergency sternotomy and closure of the wound

Table 18.1 (*cont.*)

Clinical signs include muffled heart sounds, systolic – to diastolic gradient of less then 30 mmHg, distended neck veins, and hypotension. These may be absent in hypovolemic patients	
The X-ray film may demonstrate a widening of the cardiac silhouette	
Trans-thoracic ultrasound scan is very useful	
Flail chest	**Treatment**
Common in multi-trauma patients	Patients without respiratory impairment generally do well without ventilator assistance
The injury usually occurs from direct impact	Patients with respiratory impairment require endotracheal intubation and mechanical ventilation
Crushing force from the lateral direction causes fractures in two or more sites in multiple adjacent ribs, resulting in a "floating" central portion of the chest wall	Aggressive pulmonary physiotherapy with early mobilization should be used in all patients
This results in paradoxical movement of the rest of the chest wall during respiration	Further stabilization of the chest wall may be performed by external surgical fixation
This markedly reduces the efficiency of ventilation and causes severe pain	
Crushing blow directly over the sternum with steering wheel fractures the sternum resulting in bilateral costochondral fractures and flailing of the anterior portion of the chest wall	
Chest X-ray can document multiple rib fractures	
Pulmonary contusion	**Treatment**
Potential life-threatening condition with insidious onset of symptoms	This consists of respiratory support
Patients often have other obvious injuries and detection of pulmonary contusion may escape notice	Patients may require intubation, mechanical ventilator support and antibiotic therapy
Clinical features of pulmonary contusion are: dyspnea, hypoxemia, cyanosis, tachycardia, coarse breath sounds, hemoptysis, pulmonary edema and micro-atelectasis	
The chest X-ray film may show patchy, undefined densities or homogenous consolidation	
CT scan can evaluate the extent of pulmonary contusion	
Traumatic transaction of the thoracic aortic Mortality rate = 80%	**Treatment**
Caused by acute differential deceleration injury after road traffic accidents, fall from heights or compression by heavy objects	Open surgical repair is associated with a high risk, with 30% peri-operative mortality and 8% paraplegia

(*cont.*)

Table 18.1 (*cont.*)

Most patients die at the scene of the accident	Recently, endoluminal stent-graft treatment has emerged as an alternative to conventional surgery, especially in the presence of multiple and extensive associated lesions
Survival depends on the adventitial and peri-adventitial tissues which allow for the development of a contained rupture	The procedure is carried out in the angiography suite under general anesthesia
Fractures of the scapula, first and second ribs and medial third of the clavicle should lead to a suspicion of a laceration of the thoracic aorta	
Chest X-ray can show a widening of mediastinum, right tracheal shift, elevation and rightward shift of the right bronchus, depression of the left bronchus, aortic knob outline, deviation of the esophagus to the right	
Transesophageal echocardiography is a useful diagnostic tool if available	
CT scan is mandatory	
Esophageal and diaphragmatic injury Rupture of esophagus is very rare and lethal if unrecognized	Treatment Eesophageal injury
It could present as sudden excruciating pain in the epigastrium which radiates to the chest, back or both, dyspnea, cyanosis and shock	Surgical correction when the patient is stable
Esophagoscopic visualization of localized blood in the esophagus or an actual laceration is diagnostic	Major esophageal injuries should be corrected early to reduce mediastinitis. If correction is delayed, extensive mediastinal contamination occurs
Injuries of the diaphragm are more frequent. The diagnosis is often missed	Diaphragmatic injury
Diaphragmatic injury should be suspected in any penetrating thoracic wound (gunshot, stab or accidental perforation) at or below 4th intercostal space anteriorly, 6th interspace laterally, or 8th interspace posteriorly	The treatment is always surgery by a thoracic or abdominal approach
Stomach and other abdominal viscera herniate into left thorax causing left lung collapse	The decision to repair an isolated diaphragmatic rupture in an acutely injured patient depends on how the patient tolerates the loss of normal, negative intrathoracic pressure
The clinical presentation includes dyspnea, chest or shoulder pain	Gross signs of cardiorespiratory distress or shock are indication for immediate repair
Chest X-ray may demonstrate atelectasis with silhouetting of the ipsilateral diaphragm, evidence of air-filled loops of bowel in the thorax	
Ultrasound and CT scan will confirm the diagnosis	

- Dilution of existing clotting factors from the administration of large volumes of intravenous fluids.

Infusion of a large volume of fluids is particularly detrimental in patients with pulmonary contusion and thoracic aortic disruption. In patients with thoracic aortic disruption, the medial and intimal layers are torn. The adventitia of the aorta is the only membrane that prevents aortic rupture and exsanguination. In this precarious situation, a rise in blood pressure can tear this layer resulting in sudden death.

Pulmonary contusion can cause increased capillary permeability. Tissue fluid leaks into the alveoli causing pulmonary edema. Infusions of large volumes in these cases will exacerbate the pulmonary edema. Patients with significant pulmonary contusion should receive cautious fluid boluses. The priority in managing significant thoracic hemorrhage is to control the source of bleeding as quickly as possible. The anesthetist should continually evaluate blood loss in the patient. This can be difficult to estimate directly and indirect or physiological responses to bleeding can be used such as decreasing hematocrit.

The optimal treatment of patients with hemorrhagic shock is replacement of blood volume with a combination of blood products, crystalloid and colloid intravenous fluids. Auto-transfusion techniques can be used if there is no contamination of the blood collected in the hemothorax. Cell-saver devices are used to filter and prepare the patient's blood which is then transfused back to the patient. Blood coagulopathy can develop if a large quantity of blood is auto-transfused. Transfusion of red blood cell concentrate is rarely indicated if the patient's hemoglobin is below 7 g/dL unless there is excessive ongoing blood loss. As a rule of thumb, each unit of packed red cells increases the hematocrit by approximately 3%.

Platelets transfusion is required in surgical patients when the count falls below 50×10^9 and the patient continues to bleed. Platelet transfusion of five single unit donors or one pooled unit will increase the count by 5000–10 000.

Fresh frozen plasma (FFP) is used in correcting dilution coagulopathy. Prolonged prothrombin time (PT) and partial thromboplastin time (PTT) are a useful guide to direct FFP infusion. However, processing these tests can take up to 30 minutes and patients requiring massive transfusion can receive FFP without waiting for the results.

Transfusion of cryoprecipitate is also used in correcting hemostasis. Cryoprecipitate contains factor VIII, fibrinogen, fibronectin and factor XIII. In trauma patients, consumptive coagulopathy can lead to decrease in fibrinogen levels and microvascular bleeding. Fibrinogen levels below 80–100 mg/dl are an indication for cryoprecipitate infusion.

Anesthetic considerations for emergency and urgent thoracotomy

Emergency thoracotomy is defined as thoracotomy either immediately at the site of injury or in the hospital as an integral part of the initial resuscitation process. An urgent thoracotomy is that performed at a later stage after the initial resuscitation process (Box 18.4).

Box 18.4 Indications for thoracotomy

Indications for emergency thoracotomy.
    Penetrating cardiac trauma with definitive signs of life at the scene.
    Uncontrolled life-threatening bleeding into the airway.
Indications for urgent thoracotomy.
    Open pneumothorax.
    Massive hemothorax.
    Esophageal trauma.
    Diaphragm rupture.
    Penetrating chest injury.

Emergency thoracotomy was proposed in the 1960s as an essential step in the initial resuscitation of patients in extremis with thoracic trauma. After a period of liberal use, enthusiasm for this operation faded because of its limited success. It also remained an unsuccessful operation for victims of blunt and extrathoracic trauma. However, emergency thoracotomy in the setting of cardiac tamponade from penetrating chest trauma, continues to be supported by the literature. The best chance of success is if the surgery is performed by an experienced surgeon. However, the mortality remains high.

The following are associated with a poor prognosis:

- Blunt trauma with no sign of life at the scene.
- Cardiopulmonary resuscitation for more than 10 minutes without any sign of life.
- Gunshot wound of the heart.
- Penetration of the left ventricle.
- Laceration of a coronary artery.
- Injury of one of the great vessels.
- Associated serious extrathoracic injury.
- Delayed diagnosis and treatment.

Urgent thoracotomy is also indicated in the presence of severe hemorrhage. This is defined as a blood loss of greater than 1500 ml after insertion of a chest tube drain or continued hourly blood loss of 250 ml for 3 consecutive hours. This concept was largely derived from observations made in the early 1970s based on experience predominantly with penetrating injuries. Subsequent studies have indicated that this should be applied equally to penetrating and blunt trauma.

Another indication for urgent thoracotomy is for extraction of knife blade from the chest cavity in stab injury. The blade of an embedded knife may act as a tamponade and control hemorrhage. Massive hemorrhage, hemodynamic deterioration, and possible death may result from incorrect manipulation of the knife. Embedded objects are commonly extracted under direct vision during a formal thoracotomy to ensure that no other injuries have been sustained to other vital organs. Video-assisted thoracic surgery is an important and extensively used diagnostic tool for suspected traumatic intrathoracic lesions, including stab wounds, in hemodynamically stable patients.

Anesthetic considerations

A quick standard anesthetic assessment should be performed on all trauma patients. Important information includes allergies, past medical history, previous anesthetic history and events surrounding the trauma. The anesthetic assessment of unconscious patients is difficult and can be limited to the patient's relatives and paramedical staff. All trauma patients should be considered as having a full stomach.

A reliable intravenous access should be maintained. Venous catheters inserted by the emergency team should be checked as they might have dislodged during resuscitation and transfer. Ensure that baseline blood samples for full blood count, biochemistry and blood grouping and cross-matching are sent off for analysis. In situations of massive hemorrhage, uncross-matched blood products may be required in the operating theater. Standard anesthetic monitoring should be used every time. This includes ECG, non-invasive blood pressure, SaO_2 and CO_2 analyser. Invasive monitoring of blood pressure should be considered in all these patients. It has the added advantage of providing beat-to-beat change in blood pressure and an access to measuring arterial blood gases.

All trauma patients are considered as having a full stomach. Rapid sequence induction with external cricoid pressure should be used on all patients unless contraindicated. Anesthetic agents used for intubation depend upon the patient's hemodynamic status. The technique should be tailored to avoid exacerbation of hypovolemic shock with anesthetic-induced vasodilatation.

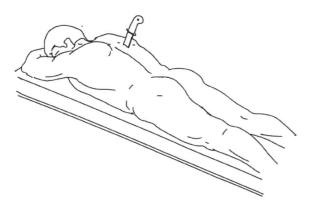

Figure 18.1 Patient with knife embedded in the posterior thorax. (*Courtesy of Mr. David Crawford.*)

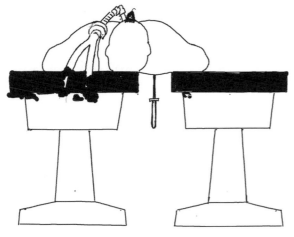

Figure 18.2 Patient positioned partially on a stretcher and an operating table with the embedded knife between them. (*Courtesy of Mr. David Crawford.*)

Patients with unknown cervical spine status should have in-line stabilization of the cervical spine during tracheal intubation. Double lumen endobronchial tubes should be used if lung separation is anticipated.

Patients with knives embedded in the back present unique difficulties with positioning for induction. The patient can be placed on his back, partially on a stretcher and partially on the operating table, the knife protruding between them. (See Figures 18.1 and 18.2.) The patient can be placed in the appropriate lateral position after induction of anesthesia.

After induction of anesthesia, the anesthetist should be attentive to the signs of pneumothorax and cardiac tamponade. These can develop insidiously during the initial resuscitation and will become life threatening when anesthesia and positive pressure ventilation are commenced. These should be excluded swiftly if the patient deteriorates after intubation.

Patients with blunt chest trauma may develop myocardial ischemia or contusions. Continuous monitoring of ECG leads 2 and V_5 is necessary to detect this. Trans-esophageal echocardiography has become useful in detecting the regional wall motion abnormalities and pericardial collections. Patients with severe lung or tracheo-bronchial trauma have a high risk of air embolism. Positive pressure ventilation should be given at the lowest possible pressures to maintain adequate oxygenation. Pain control after surgery is discussed in another chapter.

Airway management in thoracic trauma

The airway of a trauma patient should be frequently assessed as it might change. In addition to altering levels of consciousness and cardio-respiratory compromise, patients with thoracic trauma can develop expanding hematoma compressing the trachea; laryngeal fractures could result in upper airways edema. This requires anesthetic expertise.

Large subcutaneous emphysema in the neck, mediastinum or chest wall should raise the suspicion of major airway trauma. Laryngeal fractures are not common. The only indications could be hoarseness of voice in a conscious patient. Severe laryngeal trauma would require an emergency tracheotomy.

Penetrating tracheal injuries are obvious in the neck. However, blunt tracheal injuries, particularly in the unconscious patient, are difficult to diagnose. Rupture of the trachea or major bronchi is usually secondary to an injury of the chest as a result of an automobile accident. It is a serious injury with an estimated mortality of 30%. More than 80% of the ruptures of bronchi are within 2.5 cm of the carina. Injuries to the main bronchi and intrathoracic trachea are more prevalent than those to the cervical trachea because the latter is protected by the mandible and sternum anteriorly and by vertebrae posteriorly.

The clinical signs can be overlooked easily. It could present as a large pneumothorax, hemoptysis, dyspnea, subcutaneous and mediastinal emphysema. Major bronchial tears can cause a change in voice.

Bronchoscopy should be carried out promptly when tracheo-bronchial rupture is suspected, since it is the most reliable means of establishing the diagnosis.

Thoracotomy should be performed as soon as possible for surgical repair. Endotracheal intubation can exclude small tracheal injuries if the cuff is placed distal to the injury. Injuries in the distal airway require a double lumen endotracheal tube. This should be placed correctly using a FOB. Bronchial tears require double lumen endotracheal tubes and carefully placed bronchial blockers to isolate the injury and air leak.

FURTHER READING

- Bickell WH, Wall MJ Jr, Pepe PE, *et al.* Immediate versus delayed fluid resuscitation for hypotensive patients with penetrating torso injuries. *N Engl J Med* 1994; **331**: 1105–9.
- Bouillon B, Keel M, Meier C. Chest injuries – what is new? *Curr Opin Crit Care Med* 2007; **13**(6); 674–9.
- Eckert MJ, Clagett C, Martin M, *et al.* Bronchoscopy in the blast injury patient. *Arch Surg* 2006; **141**: 806–11.
- Hunt PA, Greaves I, Owens WA. Emergency thoracotomy in thoracic trauma-a review. *Injury* 2006; **37**(1): 1–19.
- Leissner KB, Ortega R, Beattie WS. Anesthesia implications of blast injury. *J Cardiothorac Vasc Anesth* 2006; **20**(6): 872–80.

Chapter 19

Pediatric thoracic procedures

TIM MURPHY AND JONATHAN HAYDEN SMITH

This chapter will deal with anesthesia for surgery to major intrathoracic structures excluding the heart and great vessels in neonates, infants and children. Compared with other pediatric surgical specialities, relatively few patients present for thoracic surgical procedures. Many of the principles which apply to both the general pediatric and the adult thoracic patient apply to pediatric thoracic anesthesia. This chapter will therefore focus on thorough pre-operative assessment, intra-operative management including techniques for one-lung ventilation (OLV) and post-operative care including analgesia as well as a brief discussion of several conditions which present specifically in the pediatric patient population.

Factors unique to the pediatric thoracic patient

There are a number of important specific considerations that apply to the pediatric population, which are discussed below.

Pediatric physiology

Significant differences between pediatric and adult physiology and anatomy include the following:

- The lungs, as organs of gas exchange, are not fully developed until at least 8 years of age.

- Children's ribs are relatively more horizontal, limiting increases in tidal volume. The diaphragm is therefore the most important muscle of respiration in a spontaneously breathing child.
- Children exhibit relatively higher basal oxygen consumption (6–8 ml/kg per min compared with 3 ml/kg per min in adults). Hypoxia develops relatively more rapidly under conditions of apnea or hypoventilation.
- Gas exchange and ventilation rapidly deteriorate during manual IPPV if the stomach is allowed to inflate with gas.
- A child's thoracic cage has relatively greater compliance (i.e. the chest wall fails to splint open the lungs). Functional residual capacity (FRC) is therefore closer to closing volume in children, predisposing to airway collapse during tidal breathing. This may increase the risk of V/Q mismatching, and therefore hypoxia, in a spontaneously breathing, anesthetized child.

One-lung ventilation in pediatric practice

Contrary to the situation in adults, when ventilation/perfusion matching may be improved with the "good lung down" position, in pediatrics V/Q matching is improved with the "good lung up." This is explained as follows:

- The more compliant thoracic cage is less able to support the dependent lung, leading to compression of dependent lung tissue.
- Because of the relationship between FRC and closing volume, airway closure may occur during ventilation with normal tidal volumes (around 7 ml/kg).
- In children, mechanical loading of the diaphragm is relatively less than adults in the lateral decubitus position. This reduces the functional advantage of the dependent diaphragm.
- Differences in lung perfusion due to the hydrostatic pressure gradient in the lateral decubitus position are relatively less in children. This reduces V/Q matching and may worsen hypoxia.

There is some evidence that in spite of these concerns, gas exchange remains entirely acceptable in children during OLV in the lateral decubitus position, particularly if a higher FiO_2 is used. Because of differences in airway management, however, some techniques for addressing hypoxia during OLV with a double lumen tube may be unavailable during pediatric OLV.

Pre-operative assessment

The anesthetist will want to know what effect the intended procedure will have on the patient's lung function in the post-operative period. Most useful techniques for making this assessment in adults – for example, spirometry, lung function testing and cardiopulmonary exercise testing – may be unavailable for younger, less cooperative children. The following should therefore be evaluated in the pre-operative visit, in addition to the standard anesthetic assessment.

- Functional capacity of the child, including symptoms of breathlessness on exercise or changes in respiratory symptoms when the child changes position.
- All data from radiological investigations, particularly including abnormalities in tracheal or mediastinal anatomy.
- Thoracic pathology is not uncommonly associated with coexistent cardiac disease. If this is suspected a cardiological opinion and an echocardiogram should be sought.
- Use of medications such as home oxygen, prophylactic antibiotics, inhaled bronchodilators or steroids, as well as data from peak flow measurements if available.
- If the patient has had previous thoracic surgery, then details of previous airway management techniques should be taken from the old anesthetic chart.
- Results of relevant hematological investigations when available. For procedures where significant blood loss is anticipated, availability of blood or blood products for transfusion should be confirmed.
- For surgical excision of malignant intrathoracic masses, a full oncological history should be sought.
- Details of relevant recent acute illnesses, in particular involving the respiratory tract.

The patient should be examined paying particular attention to the chest and heart, and a careful airway assessment completed. Oxygen saturation on air and following exercise should be available. An assessment by a physiotherapist may well provide further useful information. Finally the surgeon should be consulted as to the exact details of the intended operative procedure and any specific anesthetic technique that they may prefer.

The use of a sedating pre-medicant should be considered and individualized to each patient, although drugs which depress respiration should probably be avoided in those with particularly poor respiratory reserve.

Intra-operative management – general principles

Each phase of the anesthetic management of the pediatric thoracic patient should be carefully planned in advance and anesthetic nursing staff should be fully briefed, so that equipment is readily available. In some cases it may be advisable to have surgical staff immediately available at the time of induction of anesthesia. In addition, the following should be considered:

- Full monitoring should be established prior to induction of anesthesia. There are some younger patients for whom this may be very upsetting, in which case the absolute minimum of a pulse oximeter should be applied.
- An inhalational technique with a high inspired concentration of oxygen and sevoflurane may well be preferable, particularly for those patients in whom changes in respiratory function or airway patency may accompany induction of anesthesia. This necessitates standard monitoring of inspired and end tidal oxygen, CO_2 and anesthetic agent concentrations.
- If unavailable at the time of induction, venous access should be obtained as soon as practicable, with as large bore an intravenous canula as possible.
- Once initiated – for example following the onset of apnea or the use of muscle relaxants – manual IPPV should be as gentle as possible, using the minimum tidal volume to maintain patient oxygenation. Manual IPPV may be particularly hazardous in certain specific pathologies (see later section).
- Following securing of the airway, it may be necessary to check and recheck the position of the ET tube or blocker with a fiberoptic scope. This particularly applies when the patient is turned onto their side.
- Consideration should be given to siting an arterial line, particularly if there is anticipated

heavy blood loss, extensive or prolonged tissue resection, an expectation of the need for a period of post-operative ventilation, or if pre-operative respiratory function is poor. Similar considerations apply to the need for central venous access.

- Temperature monitoring should be available, together with techniques for warming the patient or infused fluids. Urine output monitoring may be necessary in major cases.

Techniques for OLV in pediatric patients
Deliberate endobronchial intubation

An uncut conventional endotracheal tube, half a size smaller than the predicted correct size for the patient (using the formula $4 + age/4$) is deliberately advanced into the appropriate bronchus. This is relatively easier for the right main bronchus than the left, and careful positioning of the patient's head and airway, as well as the tube and its bevel, may be necessary. The bevel is turned such that it faces the bronchus which is being intubated. If necessary a small bronchoscope (such as the 2.2 mm intubating scope) may be used to guide the tube into the appropriate bronchus and confirm its position. Scrupulous care needs to be taken while securing the tube and its position needs to be rechecked once the patient is turned onto their side. An oral airway may be useful to stabilize the tube in the patient's mouth. In a case where the right main bronchus is intubated, care needs to be taken to avoid occluding the right upper lobe bronchus. Endobronchial suction to the operated lung is not possible using this technique. It may be difficult to re-establish satisfactory two-lung ventilation (by withdrawing the tip of the tube into the main trachea) at the end of the surgical procedure owing to the inevitable leak that will follow using a relatively small ET tube. Conversely, if the tube is a good fit within the larynx, it may be difficult to achieve satisfactory deflation of the operated lung with this technique.

Double lumen cuffed endotracheal tubes

The smallest DLT available is a 26Fr (Rusch, Duluth, GA, USA), suitable for patients around 8 years of age. A left-sided 28Fr DLT (Mallinckrodt Medical, Inc., St. Louis, MO, USA) is also available for use in patients around 10 years of age.

The univent tube

This is a modified endotracheal tube (made by Fuji Systems Corporation, Tokyo, Japan) which is available in pediatric sizes down to a #3.5 mm internal diameter. There is a tracheal tube and an additional small lumen containing a bronchial blocker, which may be positioned with the help of a fiberoptic scope. The tracheal lumen of these tubes is relatively small and therefore offers high resistance to gas flow.

The endobronchial blocker

The patient's trachea is intubated with a conventional endotracheal tube of an appropriate size (Figure 19.1). An endobronchial blocker is then guided into position using a fiberoptic scope, and carefully inflated under direct vision. Various blocking devices have been used including a Fogarty embolectomy catheter, balloon-tipped radiology catheter or the Cook 5 French ('Fr') bronchial blocker (Cook Critical Care, Bloomington, IN, USA). This bronchial blocker has a channel with a Luer slip adapter that permits active deflation of the "blocked" lung by a syringe, as well as endobronchial suctioning. Great care needs to be taken in the positioning and inflation of any blocker: the balloon may herniate across the contralateral bronchial orifice, and it could cause significant or complete tracheal occlusion if it becomes displaced. It may be necessary to repeatedly recheck the position of the blocker during the course of the operation.

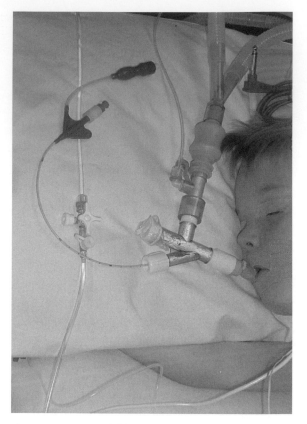

Figure 19.1 An Arndt blocker in situ for one-lung ventilation.

Choice of technique

In summary, careful pre-operative planning and good communication with the surgeon are essential. The choice of the best ventilation technique for each patient is often down to anesthetist choice, preference and experience. It is certainly the case that OLV in smaller and younger patients is technically more demanding and intrinsically prone to more complications. Two-lung ventilation is usually a perfectly acceptable and a simpler technique for many surgical procedures. To help reduce the chance of damaging the lung, apnea can be maintained while the thoracic cavity is entered. Two-lung ventilation with surgical retraction of lung tissue is generally well tolerated. V/Q matching, oxygenation and hemodynamics may well be superior while

Table 19.1 Appropriate doses for pediatric analgesia.

Opiate – intra-operative	Fentanyl bolus (up to 5 μg/kg) *OR*	Alfentanil bolus (up to 50 μg/kg) *OR*	Remifentanil infusion (up to 0.2 μg/kg per min)
Opiate – post-operative	Loading dose of morphine towards end of surgery (100–200 μg/kg)	Morphine PCA or NCA, possibly with background infusion	Codeine 1 mg/kg QDS after PCA taken down
Paracetamol	Pre-med: 30–40 mg/kg PO *OR*	Intra-operatively: 30–40 mg/kg PR or IV	Post-operatively: 90 mg/kg in 4 divided doses (for patients < 3 months of age, the dose is 60 mg/kg in 24 hours)
NSAID	Pre-med : ibuprofen 5 mg/kg PO *OR*	Intra-operatively: diclofenac 1 mg/kg PR	Post-operatively: ibuprofen 5 mg/kg TDS

both lungs remain ventilated. The disadvantage of surgical retraction of the lung is the potential for lung contusion and its sequelae of impairment of gas exchange in the post-operative period.

Peri-operative analgesia for pediatric thoracic patients

Patients will require satisfactory intra-operative and post-operative analgesia. Appropriate doses are given in Table 19.1.

- Intra-operative use of opiates is almost universal. Broadly, a combination of relatively short-acting opiates such as fentanyl, alfentanil or a remifentanil infusion, together with a loading dose of a longer-acting drug such as morphine towards the end of surgery, is reasonable.
- An appropriate loading dose of paracetamol and/or non-steroidal (such as ibuprofen) may be given as pre-medication, or given rectally after induction of anesthesia.
- Local anesthetic may be infiltrated into the wound by the surgeon, given as a post-operative infusion, or be administered by the anesthetist as a specific "block." Infusions may be given either via the paravertebral route (using a catheter sited under direct vision by the surgeon), or via the epidural route (in younger

patients it is possible to advance a caudally inserted epidural catheter towards the thoracic epidural space). The maximum bolus dose of bupivacaine is 2 mg/kg, and the infusion dose is up to 0.25 mg/kg per hour (equivalent to 0.25 ml/kg per hour of 0.1% bupivacaine solution).

Intra-operative management – specific conditions
Empyema

In the last 10 years empyema has become the commonest indication for thoracic surgery in our unit (Figure 19.2). Patients with complications of pneumonia (such as empyema or an infected para-pneumonic effusion) requiring surgical intervention constitute the largest proportion of patients presenting for thoracic surgery. Pre-operative assessment should focus on the likely need or otherwise for post-operative ventilatory support, although this may be difficult to predict. It is easier surgically to complete decortication if the diseased lung remains inflated, so OLV is not generally indicated. If pneumonia has become complicated by formation of a lung abscess, and there is concern about soiling of the contralateral lung, an OLV technique may be indicated although complete protection of the

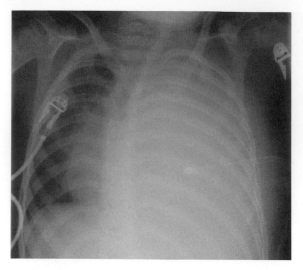

Figure 19.2 This chest X-ray shows an empyema with right shift of the mediastinum despite a chest drain in situ.

contralateral lung cannot be guaranteed with an uncuffed ET tube.

Congenital lobar emphysema (CLE), congenital cystic adenomatous malformation (CCAM), sequestrum

These relatively benign conditions represent a spectrum of abnormal development of lung tissue and present variably during the child's development, very occasionally as an emergency. Commonly the patients will have received a previous general anesthetic for CT or magnetic resonance scanning. Surgical management often involves a lobectomy. Care needs to be taken in the manual ventilation of patients with CLE, as the diseased lung segments may deflate abnormally. If over-inflated, they may compress the mediastinum and cause cardiovascular compromise.

Tracheo-esophageal fistula (TOF) repair

A detailed description of the different types of tracheo-esophageal fistula (TOF) will not be provided here, although detailed knowledge of the precise type of anatomy and a thorough pre-

operative assessment will be vital. After suctioning of the Replogle tube, anesthesia is invariably induced using an inhalational technique, and some advocate intubation during spontaneous breathing. If a relaxant is administered then avoidance of aggressive IPPV is essential, as the communication between esophagus and trachea may permit insufflation of the stomach. Additionally, lung ventilation may be impossible if the fistula is large and it is therefore easier for gases to go into the (low resistance to flow) stomach than the lung. The tip of the ET tube needs to be positioned to occlude the fistula, and careful auscultation of the lungs is required to achieve this. Alternatively, it may be necessary to intubate the contralateral bronchus and utilize OLV until the fistula is repaired. The anesthetist needs to be vigilant during surgical manipulation of the fistula, as airway obstruction may occur. Although a period of care on an ITU or HDU may be preferable post-operatively, ventilation is not mandatory. Analgesia is commonly provided via an epidural infusion.

Congenital diaphragmatic hernia (CDH)

This condition is associated with a relatively high mortality, mainly from associated pathology such as ipsilateral (or bilateral) pulmonary hypoplasia and pulmonary hypertension. Patients may present for surgery having been intubated and stabilized shortly after birth; this may involve use of pulmonary vasodilators, oscillatory ventilation or even ECMO. Surgical repair is commonly performed via a laparotomy incision. If intubation is necessary pre-operatively, a technique that avoids gastrointestinal distension (from manual IPPV) is vital. Perioperative measures to maintain physiological stability and minimize PVR (hypocapnia, alkalosis and a satisfactory PaO_2), together with the avoidance of lung barotrauma, are both necessary. A period of post-operative ventilation is almost invariable, avoiding the need for an anesthetic technique that incorporates extubation at the end of surgery.

Malignancy

Fortunately, tumors of the lung and mediastinum are relatively uncommon in pediatric anesthetic practice. Surgical removal of lung tumors (whether primary or secondary) is generally easier if an OLV technique is employed. Particular attention must, however, be paid to patients presenting for biopsy of a suspected malignant mediastinal tumor. These patients, in addition to cardiovascular compromise from compression of vascular structures, may have respiratory symptoms (particularly worryingly, orthopnea) due to airway compression. More importantly they may develop *intractable* airway obstruction after induction of anesthesia. It may therefore be preferable to complete some of the chemotherapy cycles before attempting to obtain tumor tissue for definitive biopsy. For patients presenting for anesthesia with SVC obstruction, it is advisable to site an intravenous cannula in a peripheral vein that drains into the IVC.

Bronchogenic cyst

Bronchogenic cysts may occur throughout the tracheobronchial tree and are often fluid-filled. Management of these lesions almost invariably involves surgical excision, during which OLV is frequently necessary.

Bronchoscopy/bronchography

General anesthesia for bronchoscopy invariably utilizses a spontaneously breathing technique with sevoflurane, and is commonly performed as a day case procedure. After induction of anesthesia it is common to spray the vocal cords with lignocaine to prevent coughing or laryngospasm during insertion of the bronchoscope. Alternatively the bronchoscopist may use a "spray-as-you-go" technique. An intravenous antisialogogue (atropine 20 µg/kg or glycopyrrolate 10 µg/kg) may be useful. When the vocal cords have been sprayed it is mandatory to observe a period of 1–2 hours nil-by-mouth post-operatively. Anesthesia for bronchography is commonly associated with the need to investigate suspected tracheobronchomalacia (TBM). Patients commonly present with difficulty to wean from mechanical ventilation together with any pathology associated with TBM such as left atrial enlargement. General anesthesia (invariably an intravenous technique) with a mechanically supported mode of spontaneous breathing is the technique of choice, particularly as, with a sophisticated ventilator, it may be possible to define accurately the pressure necessary to maintain tracheobronchial patency throughout the respiratory cycle. One technique for injecting contrast into the tracheobronchial tree utilizes an epidural catheter, which passes through a suitable airtight adaptor attached to the patient's ET tube.

Foreign body removal

Patients commonly present as an emergency for removal of an inhaled foreign body although the history may occasionally precede the presentation at hospital by several days. Traditionally anesthesia is induced using an inhalational technique in order to maintain spontaneous respiration, which theoretically prevents the foreign body from being pushed further into the patient's lungs during positive pressure ventilation. In practice, a cautious intravenous technique with spontaneous respiration may be equally satisfactory. Anesthetic management requires very close cooperation between surgeon and anesthetist: invariably the surgeon utilizes a rigid ventilating bronchoscope to visualize the foreign body. Using a suitable adaptor, a simple Ayre's T-piece (with or without an open-ended reservoir bag) can be attached to the bronchoscope to maintain inhalational anesthesia and oxygenation until the foreign body has been removed.

Tracheal surgery

Any tracheal surgical procedure is likely to result in a "shared airway" and therefore require close cooperation and planning between surgeon and anesthetist. Extensive distal tracheal surgery may require the use of cardiopulmonary bypass.

Post-operative care

Aside from the provision of adequate analgesia (and daily input from the acute pain service), it is important to ensure that pediatric thoracic patients are nursed in an appropriate post-operative environment, which includes facilities for the provision of supplemental humidified oxygen, physiotherapy, and monitoring of oxygen saturation and respiratory rate as a minimum standard. As discussed above, certain patients will require a ventilated intensive care bed post-operatively.

Summary

Providing satisfactory peri-operative management of the pediatric thoracic patient requires the highest standards of pre-operative assessment, technical expertise and communication between team members, but is both challenging and rewarding.

FURTHER READING

- Golianu B, Hammer GB. Pain management for paediatric thoracic surgery. *Curr Opin Anaesthes* 2005; **18**: 5–11.
- Hammer GB. Paediatric thoracic surgery. *Anesth Analges* 2001; **92**: 1449–64.
- Haynes SR, Bonner S. Anaesthesia for thoracic surgery in children. *Paediatr Anaesth* 2000; **10**: 237–51.
- Tobias JD. Thoracic surgery in children. *Curr Opin Anaesthes* 2001; **14**: 77–85.

Chapter 20

Significance of age in practice of thoracic anesthesia

VIJAY JEGANATH AND JAYANTA NANDI

Effect of age on thoracic anesthesia

The population in the developed world is aging, together with an increasing life expectancy for both men and women. The attitude towards treating diseases in the elderly has therefore changed in favor of obtaining not only symptomatic improvement in quality of life, but also survival benefit and even definitive cure. In the UK, at present, there are more people in their 70s and 80s than ever before. A recent American survey noted that the number of septuagenarians has tripled; octogenarians – being now the fastest expanding population group – have increased 10-fold in some surgical practices, over the past two decades.

The incidence of thoracic pathologies in the elderly of the developed world is also rising. Worldwide, lung cancer is the most common cancer with around 1.3 million new cases diagnosed every year. The bulk of thoracic surgical work in Europe and the USA is related to resection of lung cancer. In the UK, in spite of having about 37 700 cases diagnosed each year (second commonest cancer in UK), fewer than 4000 (under 10%) of cases are resected – a stark contrast to resection rates of 24% and 25% reported in Dutch and American patients. This difference is amplified in elderly patients who are much less likely to have surgery for lung cancer in the UK than their counterparts in Europe and America. The British Thoracic Society and The Society of Cardiothoracic Surgeons of Great Britain and Ireland (SCTS) are rallying the need for doubling lung cancer operations and specialist thoracic surgeons in the UK. The workload of thoracic anesthetists, like their thoracic surgical colleagues, is expected to increase with a higher proportion of patients being over 65 years of age. This group of patients is also more likely to undergo VATS procedures.

Aging is a complex process that results in a decreased capacity for adaptation and produces a gradual reduction in functional reserve in many of the body's organ systems. In the absence of comorbidity, physical age (and quality of tissues) together with physiologic age (especially response to exercise) is more important than chronological age to determine a favorable outcome following anesthetic and surgical procedures in thoracic surgery.

Advanced age is not a disease but increases the likelihood of age-related diseases. The mortality data from the UK Office of National Statistics indicate that, for age over 65, circulatory diseases are the most common cause of death (accounting for 40%). Pneumonia as a cause of death also increases with age to account for one in ten deaths among those aged 85 and over (deaths

Core Topics in Thoracic Anesthesia, ed. Cait P. Searl and Sameena T. Ahmed. Published by Cambridge University Press.
© Cambridge University Press 2009.

from respiratory causes constitute 13–17% in this group). This indirectly reflects the organ systems that are commonly affected by age-related reduction in physiologic reserve – that may be compounded by disease – and are consequently likely to struggle when exposed to the stresses of anesthesia and surgery with their associated potential complications (Box 20.1).

Age and the risk–benefit equation in thoracic anesthesia and surgery

The success of a procedure in thoracic surgery – and hence the decision to offer the option – is justified by the favorable outcome following the procedure. This is weighed formulating the risk–benefit equation. A major decision-making step relates to identifying the group of patients who are most likely to obtain symptomatic (improved quality of life) and prognostic (increased survival and possibly curative) benefit with the least risk. The risks encompass mortality, morbidity, quality of life and long-term survival issues. They have to be acceptable to both the healthcare provider and the patient.

As in other fields, risk outcomes are measured in thoracic procedures using the parameters of mortality, morbidity and potential for adverse effects on quality of life.

Mortality associated with anesthesia and surgery for thoracic pathologies is defined as the death rate within 30 days following the procedure. Historically, advanced age (over 70 years) and very old age (over 80 years) were associated with poorer outcome in terms of early (30-day) mortality and morbidity. It is generally recognized that the elderly with comorbidities have worse outcomes than those without. There is currently no definite widely accepted risk-scoring model in thoracic surgery to quantify advancing age as a predictor of outcome – as there is for some cardiac surgical procedures (e.g. Parsonnet score from North America; EUROscore for European populations).

Recent results confirm that anesthetic and surgical mortality and morbidity in the elderly undergoing thoracic procedures is decreasing. Although the reasons are multifactorial, improvements in technology, expertise, experience in patient and procedure selection and anesthetic, surgical and peri-operative care have a major role to play. The challenge lies in dealing with the elderly patients with comorbidities.

Age in itself is not a contraindication for anesthesia in thoracic surgery. In fact there are no absolute contraindications of general anesthesia in the elderly undergoing thoracic surgery. It is generally believed that if the patient is fit enough to tolerate a thoracic surgical procedure, they are fit enough to tolerate anesthesia for it! The main cautions of thoracic anesthesia in the elderly are those of geriatric anesthesia in general and those of the surgical procedure itself.

In the elderly, risk assessment should focus on identifying the physiologic state and reserve of specific organ systems. It is often more challenging to identify previously undiagnosed comorbidity, optimize it and try to predict its bearing on the outcome. This is often compounded by the difficult decision of tailoring the appropriate procedure with aims of obtaining more extensive but curative resections over a less stressful, more limited (hence likely palliative) procedure.

The necessity of a meticulous pre-anesthetic and pre-operative work up cannot be overemphasized.

Pre-anesthetic assessment

The pre-operative evaluation of an elderly patient is best accomplished several days before the surgery and after all information has been obtained from the surgeon or primary care physician. The assessment includes a history, physical examination and review of the medical information. Laboratory testing is indicated by comorbid conditions and the type of surgery contemplated. The aim is to detect and optimize comorbidities and quantify

Box 20.1 Age and pathophysiology

Cardiovascular physiology

The cardiac output falls by 1% per year, beginning at age of 30 years.

The maximum rate of oxygen use (VO_2 max) declines steadily at 10% per decade and halves between the ages of 20 and 80 years.

Endothelial changes throughout the vascular tree lead to stiffening of the vascular wall, reduced compliance and consequently increased peripheral vascular resistance.

The ventricle remains stiff during phases of diastolic filling which reduces end diastolic volume and cardiac output.

Predisposition to ischemic heart disease.

Predisposes to atrial arrhythmias.

Reduced SA node automaticity and beta-adrenergic receptor responsiveness causes a reduction in the maximum attainable heart rate.

Decreased baroreceptor sensitivity causing reduced baroreflex-mediated heart rate increase to compensate for hypotension.

Pulmonary physiology

Forced expiratory volume in 1 second (FEV_1) progressively declines with aging resulting in an FEV_1:VC ratio < 70% by age 70 years.

Dead space ventilation can double between the ages of 20 and 65 years old. Ventilation-perfusion mismatching leads to decreased oxygen transfer with increased alveolar-arterial oxygen gradient.

Impaired chest wall movement from joint stiffening of chest wall, inspiratory muscle atrophy and loss of elastic recoil of lung reduce intrathoracic volumes and vital capacity with age.

Loss of parenchymal elasticity and early small airway collapse change gas flow characteristics. Impaired elasticity causes air trapping and thickened parenchyma causes increased closure volume of small airways predisposing to collapse.

Additionally, aging causes decreased responsiveness to hypercapnia and hypoxia due to decreased carotid and aortic body sensitivities.

The sum of the respiratory changes associated with aging ultimately increases work of breathing, reduces efficiency of oxygenation and limits the maximal breathing capacity by age 70 years to 50% of that at age 30 years.

Renal physiology

Renal functions reduce about 1% per year beyond age 30.

Age-related atrophy of the parenchyma and sclerotic change of the vasculature cause glomerulosclerosis with a progressive reduction in functional renal mass impairing creatinine clearance.

The age-related decline in cardiac output impacts renal plasma flow and glomerular filtration rate.

Gastrointestinal changes

Decreased hepatic function, increased gastric acidity and altered absorption.

Nervous system changes

Brain atrophic changes including neuronal death.

Decrease in norepinephrine and dopamine synthesis.

Decreased autonomic responsiveness.

Orthostatic hypotension.

Thermoregulation with increased heat loss and reduced heat tolerance. The elderly are vulnerable to hypothermia and its consequences.

(cont.)

Box 20.1 *(cont.)*

Nutrition

Malnutrition is often underestimated in the elderly.

Inability to self-care due to mental or physical problems, inadequate social support, concomitant bowel disturbances and poor dietary habits predispose to the problem.

In a recent UK series more than 40% of patients undergoing lung resection had a body mass index and skin fold thickness below the 25th centile.

Pharmacologic milieu

Loss of skeletal muscle (lean body mass), increase in percentage of body fat (more in women) and up to a 20–30% reduction in circulating blood volume occurs by age 75.

A decrease in total body water leads to higher peak drug concentrations after bolus or rapid infusion.

Protein binding of anesthetic drugs is less efficient causing exaggerated pharmacologic effects.

Decreased cardiac output and lower tissue perfusion can delay the time-to-peak effect.

Prolong drug duration of action by slowing metabolism and excretion.

Increased percentage of body fat results in an increased availability of lipid storage sites and a greater reservoir for sequestration of lipid-soluble anesthetic agents, thus prolonging their action.

---

objectively the extent of reduced physiologic reserve of systems. The difficulty remains in discriminating clearly between changes due to aging itself and the consequences of age-related disease.

Screening for cardiovascular comorbidities

The incidence of smoking and age-related atherosclerotic cardiovascular disease is high in the thoracic surgical population. Eighty percent of patients older than 80 years have identifiable cardiovascular disease including hypertension, coronary disease, peripheral vascular disease, congestive heart failure (CHF) as well as arrhythmia. Atrial fibrillation is the most common arrhythmia, estimated to be present in 10% of patients over 80 years old. Over the age of 65 years, congestive heart failure is present in 10% of individuals, and is a leading cause of post-operative morbidity and mortality after surgical procedures.

Estimation of cardiac reserve

Most elderly patients with cardiac dysfunction are compensated and will show signs of disease only

when stressed. Physical reserve of elderly patients is difficult to estimate under circumstances of a sedentary lifestyle or general debility. The Goldman Multifactorial risk index and the American Heart Association/American College of Cardiology practice guidelines provide some direction to working up the cardiovascular systems to predict cardiovascular risk in non-cardiac surgery and are equally applicable to the elderly.

Screening for pulmonary comorbidities

The age-related exposure to environmental changes and consequent prevalence of underlying smoking-related and occupational lung disease adds to the comorbidity. Chronic obstructive pulmonary disease (COPD) is the primary diagnosis in 18% of all hospital admissions in patients older than 65 years. The death rate for COPD has increased by 70% over the last three decades. With early diagnosis and aggressive pre-operative pulmonary treatment, complication rates in the elderly with COPD can be minimized.

Pulmonary evaluation

Predicting pulmonary recovery relies on formal pulmonary function testing with both volume and flow studies and assessment of exercise capability and reserve.

It has been shown that achieving an exercise capacity of only 2 minutes with a heart rate of 99 beats per minute can lower an elderly patient's complication rate from 42% to 9% and mortality rate from 7% to 1%. A VO_2max < 60% is an independent risk factor associated with higher cardiopulmonary morbidity and mortality after pulmonary resection. The British Thoracic Society (BTS) recommendations for evaluation of thoracic patients undergoing lung resections provide useful guidance. The importance of correctly predicting the post-operative values of lung function cannot be overemphasized.

Renal evaluation

Cardiopulmonary functional reserve can be quantified and assessed clinically using various exercise or maximal stress tests. However, there is at present no comparable approach to assessment of renal, hepatic, immune or nervous system functional reserve. Reduced skeletal muscle mass may make serum creatinine a less sensitive indicator of renal functional impairment in the elderly. Calculated creatinine clearance remains the most sensitive marker of renal function in the elderly. Need for dialysis support in renal failure has a considerable impact on outcomes and consequently the decision to operate in elderly patients with thoracic problems.

Nutritional evaluation

Gastrointestinal problems have a bearing on the nutritional state of the elderly awaiting thoracic procedures. This highlights the need to be aware of problems like: hepatic cirrhosis, constipation, fecal impaction, fecal incontinence, osteoporosis or vitamin B_{12} deficiency due to poor absorption.

Albumin, a marker of nutritional status, may serve as a surrogate marker for the pre-operative health status of the surgical geriatric patient.

Neurological evaluation

Accurate evaluation of pre-operative state forms a baseline to identify procedural neurological morbidity, formulate rehabilitation goals and estimate quality of life post-operatively. Small vessel changes in the brain and cerebral atrophy with consequent undiagnosed cognitive impairment and dementia is common in the elderly.

Age-related diseases such as cerebral arteriosclerosis, Alzheimer's and Parkinson's disease are all more common with advancing age. Most strokes affect those older than 70 years and the risk doubles every 10 years after age 55. There are also age-related psychiatric disorders. The symptoms are often depression, dementia, confusion, catatonia and delirium.

Response to general anesthesia

There is a general perception that the elderly have a larger decrease in blood pressure at a given concentration of a volatile anesthetic than younger patients. The evidence to support this common observation is generally lacking. The required minimum alveolar concentration (MAC) for inhalational agents decreases linearly with patient age. The reduced total anesthetic requirement for geriatric patients also applies to local anesthetics, narcotics, barbiturates, benzodiazepines and other intravenous anesthetic agents (Box 20.2, Table 20.1).

Long-term systemic hypertension alters cerebral autoregulation and necessitates higher systemic blood pressures peri-operatively in the hypertensive elderly. Reduction of vascular tone from the vasodilatory effects of anesthetic agents, for example, may decrease coronary blood flow leading to

Table 20.1 Choice of anesthetic agent.

Thiopental:	Decreased baroreceptor reflex and increased vascular wall rigidity can cause a dangerous drop in blood pressure
Ketamine	Stimulates the cardiovascular system, beneficial in hypovolemic patients, disadvantageous in patients with ischemic heart disease
	When used in combination with a benzodiazepine, the cardiovascular stimulation will be attenuated
	Ketamine increases airway secretions
Etomidate	Good choice for inducing anesthesia in the hemodynamically tenuous elderly because it possesses less cardiovascular depression than the barbiturates
Propofol	Produces dose-dependent cardiovascular and respiratory depression
	Effects can be minimized if propofol is injected slowly
	There is an age-related decrease in propofol clearance, resulting in a decreased maintenance dose
	Propofol is a good choice for many elderly patients because it offers quick recovery with few side effects
	Patients older than 80 exhibit less post-anesthetic mental impairment with propofol compared with other agents

Box 20.2 General anesthetic precautions for the elderly

Difficult neck anatomy for intubation including increased limitation of neck mobility from arthritis should be suspected and identified pre-operatively.

Care during positioning and moving elderly patients. This is helped by prior knowledge of arthritic, painful, stiff or prosthetic joints.

Calculation of appropriate doses of opiates, analgesics, anesthetic agents taking into account the pharmacokinetic and pharmacodynamic effects in the elderly.

Optimum hydration and strict fluid balance management.

ischemia and consequently uncover the limited cardiac reserve of a patient. Development of atrial fibrillation can remove the atrial contraction (or kick) and lead to reduced end diastolic volume and cardiac output.

Outcomes: specific procedure-related mortality and morbidity
Pulmonary resections

More than 40% of all patients with lung cancer presenting in the UK are aged over 75 years and efforts are in progress to improve resection rates and outcomes in this age group.

With approximately 33 000 deaths each year in the UK, lung cancer has an enormous impact on national mortality and currently accounts for 6% of all deaths and 22% of all deaths from cancer in the UK, being the most common cause of death from cancer for both men and women. Three-quarters of all deaths from lung cancer occur in people aged 65 and over.

Older studies quoted mortality rates after resection in elderly patients of up to 15–20% but more recent data suggest rates of 4–10%. Age has no significant effect on mortality up to 80 years. As in younger patients, studies in the elderly have shown that mortality is increased after pneumonectomy – especially right pneumonectomy – compared with lobectomy. In the elderly, mortality rates from reported series average 14% (range 6–36%) for pneumonectomy compared with 4–7% for lobectomy. However, these differences diminish if patients are very carefully selected with attention to comorbidity. Mortality following resection at any age should not be in excess of 4% for lobectomy and 8% for pneumonectomy.

British Thoracic Society recommendations:

1. Peri-operative morbidity increases with advancing age. Elderly patients undergoing lung resection are more likely to require intensive peri-operative support. Pre-operatively, a careful assessment of comorbidity needs to be made.

2. Surgery for stage I and II disease can be as effective in patients over 70 years as in younger patients. Such patients should be considered for surgical treatment regardless of age.

3. Age over 80 alone is not a contraindication to lobectomy or wedge resection for stage I disease. Pneumonectomy is associated with a higher mortality risk in the elderly. Age should be a factor in deciding suitability for pneumonectomy.

MORBIDITY

The Lung Cancer Study Group report found no significant difference between morbidity rates between lobectomy (28.2%) and pneumonectomy (31.9%). Continuous monitoring capabilities, improved cardiovascular pharmacotherapies and gentle mechanical ventilation strategies have played a role. Pulmonary artery pressure monitoring is beneficial in select patients with cardiopulmonary comorbidities.

Esophageal resections

Esophageal resection is the standard treatment of both squamous cell cancers and adenocarcinomas of the esophagus. It is essentially a disease of older age, with two-thirds of cases being diagnosed over 65 years of age.

Improvements in patient selection, anesthesia, operative technique, and peri-operative care have dramatically reduced operative mortality over the past 20 years. Pre-operative risk analysis has been shown to cause a reduction in post-operative mortality from 9.4% to 1.6% (all ages) and is equally applicable for the elderly. A team-based approach produces a significant decrease in the mortality of esophagectomy over time. Mortality results in UK for 2001 were 7%.

For patients with esophageal cancer, Naunheim *et al.* showed that age alone is independent risk factor for poor outcomes. Patients over 70 years old tend to have a higher mortality rate after esophagectomy when compared with younger patients. Minimally invasive esophagectomy holds the potential for further reducing operative morbidity and mortality. No prospective trials have directly compared traditional open esophagectomy with minimally invasive surgery among elderly patients.

Neurocognitive dysfunction after elderly thoracic surgery

Advanced age is an independent risk factor for postoperative cognitive dysfunction (POCD). Incidence in the elderly varies widely from 1–61% and its cause is believed to be multifactorial. In a large multinational study in the elderly (above 60 years), POCD was present in 25.8% of patients 1 week after surgery and in 9.9% of patients 3 months after surgery. This was compared with a control group of hospitalized patients not undergoing surgery who had a POCD rate of 3.4% 1 week after hospitalization and 2.8% 3 months after hospitalization. Risk factors for early dysfunction include pre-operative severe illness, impaired cognitive functioning, physical debilitation, history of dementia, increasing age, duration of anesthesia, a second operation, post-operative infections and respiratory complications. The only risk factor for the longer-term decline that achieved statistical significance was age. Transient hypoxia, hypotension and anesthetic technique did not appear to be independent risk factors. Recent findings suggest that post-operative cognitive dysfunction may persist at least 3 months after otherwise uncomplicated surgery.

Treatment should focus on identifying and treating organic causes, including electrolyte abnormalities, hypoxemia, pain, sepsis, dehydration and malnutrition. Prevention provides the most effective strategy for lowering the incidence. Protocols that provide cognitive stimulation, adequate sleep, early mobilization and reduce sensory deficit have been shown to lower the incidence. Education of patients and family are key issues. Supportive care should be administered to provide the best chance for recovery. Many of these patients lose their ability to live independently and are ultimately discharged to long-term care facilities.

End-of-life issues

Most patients would rather maintain an independent lifestyle rather than gain a few months or years of life in a debilitated state. When assessing the risk–benefit ratio for an elderly patient, the predicted life expectancy of the patient and quality of life after intervention must be considered. The patient should be aware of the specific risks related to a patient's age and comorbidities and the potential need for rehabilitation services or nursing home care post-operatively. Patients should be encouraged to take control of end-of-life decisions and relieve the burden from their families by establishing an advanced directive to physicians outlining the care they desire.

Conclusion

Greater numbers of over 75s are now presenting with bigger challenges to the thoracic surgical speciality. The goalposts of healthcare delivery standards have been moved with expectations of better results following anesthesia and surgery in thoracic surgery in the elderly. The improvement in technology and expertise development in this subgroup stretches the speciality and has a beneficial effect on peri-operative care delivery in thoracic surgery in all age-groups on the whole.

The challenge for the future will be to strike an optimum balance between best-available and most cost-effective options of treating the elderly thoracic patient. This is in the light of the increasing per capita healthcare costs devoted to this expanding age group.

FURTHER READING

- The Critical Underprovision of Thoracic Surgery in the UK. accessed @ http://www.scts.org/doc/6168. 30 January 2002.
- British Thoracic Society and Society of Cardiothoracic Surgeons of Great Britain & Ireland Working Party. Guidelines on the selection of patients with lung cancer for surgery. *Thorax* 2001; **56**: 89–108.
- Loran DB, Zwischenberger JB. Thoracic surgery in the elderly. *J Am Coll Surg* 2004; **199**: 773–84.
- Naunheim KS, Hanosh J, Zwischenberger J, *et al.* Esophagectomy in the septuagenarian. *Ann Thorac Surg* 1993; **56**: 880–4.

Chapter 21

Management of the morbidly obese patient

SAMEENA T. AHMED

Morbid obesity refers to those with a body mass index (BMI) greater than 40, or than 35 kg/m^2 in the presence of obesity-related comorbidity.

The prevalence of obesity is increasing, with about one-third of the population of industrialized countries being at least 20% overweight. This trend is just as apparent in the UK as elsewhere. The International Obesity Task Force, a non-government organization that studies the obesity epidemic, estimates that one out of every five people worldwide is overweight or obese. Obesity, defined as a BMI higher than 30, has increased from 8% to 30% of the population in the USA since 1994. It has also been estimated that age-adjusted morbid obesity, defined as a BMI greater than 40, has increased from 2.9% to 4.7%. As a result, increasing numbers of obese patients are scheduled for every type of surgical procedure, including thoracic operations. The increased mortality rate associated with morbid obesity has been appreciated since the time of Hippocrates who wrote in his Aphorisms that "those naturally fat are more liable to sudden death than the thin."

Since obesity is a chronic condition, a potential risk reduction is possible with weight reduction programs. These include behavior modifications, exercise and diet. However, few patients are successful in reducing their weight pre-operatively, although some evidence suggests that patients generally have better recovery and increased mobility with major surgical procedures after pre-operative weight reduction. Starvation or low calorie intake may be dangerous and lead to cardiac arrhythmias or sudden death. Patients who have previously had bariatric surgery may have latent malnutrition due to malabsorption.

Safe and successful treatment of the morbidly obese patient requires a level of organizational commitment, protocols, expertise and staff training. The Association of Anaesthetists of Great Britain and Ireland have published guidelines on peri-operative management of morbidly obese patients.

Although obese patients comprise an ever-increasing percentage of thoracic surgical patients, current anesthetic management is based on experience with morbidly obese patients undergoing other surgical procedures. Morbid obesity in itself is not a contraindication to thoracic surgery. Given the potential problems of extreme obesity, there is a need for clinical studies to develop anesthetic management strategies for morbidly obese thoracic surgical patients.

Pre-operative assessment

All patients should have their height and weight measured and BMI calculated. Patients with morbid obesity should be identified by the surgeons and referred to the anesthetists at an earlier stage for pre-operative assessment. Successful outcome could depend upon having appropriate hospital equipment (operating table, bed, hoist etc.) at a hospital that does not have facilities for routine bariatric surgery.

Patients undergoing thoracic surgery with excessive BMI are likely to have other comorbid factors including the five obesity-related illnesses:

- Type II diabetes mellitus.
- Hypertension.
- Hyperlipidemia.
- Stroke.
- Coronary artery disease.

These illnesses account for approximately 85% of the increased health problems and economic burden of obesity. The risk of ischemic stroke in the obese is twice as high as the normal population.

Cardiovascular system

The pathophysiology of cardiovascular disease related to obesity involves an increase in both pre-load and after-load. There is an increase in pre-load as approximately 3 ml of blood volume are needed per 100 g of adipose tissue. Increased blood volume increases pre-load, stroke volume, cardiac output and myocardial work. This increases the levels of catecholamines, mineralocorticoids, renin and aldosterone which can increase after-load. This results in ventricular hypertrophy, decreased compliance, diastolic dysfunction and eventually ventricular failure ensues. Sudden death from cardiac arrhythmias or sinus arrest can occur. The diastolic dysfunction characteristic of obesity results in poor fluid tolerance.

Non-invasive blood pressure monitoring by cuff sphygmomanometer is often inaccurate due to size discrepancy; therefore, an indwelling arterial catheter should be employed when hemodynamic stability is in question.

Morbidly obese patients also have a greater risk of pulmonary hypertension due to obstructive sleep apnea and CO_2 retention. In longstanding cases, this can cause right-ventricular hypertrophy and eventually right heart failure. Even asymptomatic obese patients have some degree of right-ventricular dysfunction which can be demonstrated by echocardiography. Similarly, systemic hypertension with left ventricular hypertrophy can eventually cause left heart failure (obesity cardiomyopathy). The presence of angina or other cardiac symptoms requires a more thorough cardiac evaluation.

A careful history and examination may reveal signs and symptoms of cardiac disease, but may also be limited by the patient's exercise tolerance. Pharmacologic stress testing should be considered for patients who are unable to exercise sufficiently.

Pulmonary system

The pathophysiology of respiratory insufficiency associated with excessive weight was initially studied by Burwell in 1956. They coined the term "Pickwickian syndrome" to describe a markedly obese patient who fell asleep in a poker game while holding a hand containing three aces and two kings. Obesity results in a restrictive lung pattern due to both increased pulmonary blood volume and increased chest wall mass from adipose tissue. Abnormal diaphragm position, upper airway resistance and increased daily CO_2 production exacerbate respiratory load and further increase the work of breathing. The consequences of this restrictive pattern are decreased functional residual capacity, vital capacity, total lung capacity, inspiratory capacity, minute ventilatory volume and expiratory reserve volume. Morbidly obese patients with asthma or COPD are at a greater risk of postoperative complications. Patients with a wheeze may have early airway closure rather than asthma.

Patients may also exhibit an obesity-related obstructive air flow pathology that manifests itself as an increased ratio of forced expiratory volume in 1 s to forced vital capacity (FEV_1: FVC).

Spirometry usually reveals a restrictive defect with decreases in expiratory reserve volume and functional residual volume with associated small-airway collapse during tidal breathing. These changes result in ventilation/perfusion (V/Q) mismatch, an elevated shunt fraction and relative hypoxemia. At present, there are no studies to determine predictive baseline spirometry in the morbidly obese patients. However, studies have demonstrated that post-operative values for FEV_1 and forced vital capacity decrease proportionally as BMI increases. Therefore, it is likely that morbidly obese patients experience greater reductions in pulmonary function following thoracic operations.

Obstructive sleep apnea

Obesity is strongly correlated with obstructive sleep apnea syndrome (OSA). This condition is characterized by repetitive partial or complete obstruction of the upper airway associated with arterial blood oxygen desaturation and arousal from sleep. Associated symptoms include snoring, systemic and pulmonary hypertension, nocturnal angina, sleep-related cardiac dysrhythmias, insomnia and daytime somnolence. The suspicion is further increased if the patient has a large neck (circumference > 40 cm) with adipose tissue in the neck. Moderate to severe OSA may be present in more than half the morbidly obese population. Unfortunately most morbidly obese surgical patients may not have had a sleep study to confirm the diagnosis and it may not be practical, depending on the urgency of surgery. This has important implications for airway management and the use of sedatives and opiates in the peri-operative period. All morbidly obese patients should be presumed to have OSA and managed within that context.

These patients may be on home ventilatory support via CPAP or non-invasive ventilation systems which should be available for post-operative use. The home ventilation system can be limited by the amount of oxygen they deliver.

Airway assessment

A morbidly obese patient, especially with a history or symptoms suggestive of OSA, may have a diminution of the pharyngeal space secondary to fat deposition in the pharyngeal wall, which can make airway access and mask ventilation difficult. Intubation may be made more difficult because of the presence of a fat pad at the back of the neck, or because of deposition of fat into the soft tissues of the breast in women. Brodsky et al. found that a Mallampatti score of III or IV and increased neck circumference are predictors of potential difficulty with tracheal intubation in a morbidly obese patient. Unlike patients with COPD, most morbidly obese patients tend to have a normal size trachea. It is worth examining the chest X-rays and CT scans to determine the tracheo-bronchial anatomy and airway diameters.

Nutrition and metabolism

Despite their weight, morbidly obese patients may have a poor nutritional status. Obese patients have an increased resting energy requirement due to increased BMI. Central adipose tissues are more metabolically active than the peripheral adipose tissues. Obesity is characterized by the "metabolic X syndrome" with insulin resistance, hyperinsulinemia, hyperglycemia, coronary artery disease, hypertension and hyperlipidemia. Substrate overload leads to baseline resistance to insulin with chronically elevated serum levels of insulin. Elevated basal insulin concentrations in obesity suppresses lipid mobilization from body stores, causing accelerated proteolysis to support gluconeogenesis, which in turn forces rapid loss of muscle mass and early deconditioning. "Starving" morbidly obese patients

147

Box 21.1 Organ system pathology

Respiratory:	↓ FRC, TLC, VC, inspiratory capacity and expiratory reserve volume. Obstructive sleep apnea syndrome
Cardiovascular:	↑ Blood volume and vascular tone, ↓ ventricular contractility
Renal:	Hypertensive and diabetic nephropathy
Hematologic:	↑ Fibrinogen, ↓ AT-III venous stasis, impaired neutrophil function
Gastrointestinal:	Tendency for hiatus hernia, ↑ Gastric secretion volume and GERD
Metabolic:	↑ Resting energy expenditure, Insulin resistance ↑ Proteolysis

during the peri-operative period is erroneous (Box 21.1).

Risk reduction strategies in the peri-operative period

Appropriate risk reduction strategies should be considered at each stage of the patient's journey in the hospital from outpatient assessment through to inpatient admission, operating theater, high dependency and ward. Special equipment may be required such as beds, operating table, hoists etc. to accommodate the morbidly obese patient. All hospital equipment should have maximum weight restrictions clearly displayed. Specialized electrical beds that can enable patients to be raised without need for manual handling would be ideal. Medical and nursing staff looking after these patients should regularly receive training on lifting and handling morbidly obese patients. Patients should be encouraged to move themselves whenever possible.

Induction of anesthesia

Sedative pre-medication with benzodiazepines and opiates can have prolonged effects. In patients with OSA, they increase the risk of respiratory depression and are best avoided. Patients with gastro-esophageal reflux should have antacid prophylaxis and a proton pump inhibitor if there are no contraindications.

The standard physiological monitoring should be established prior to induction of anesthesia.

It may be difficult to measure the patient's blood pressure accurately using an upper arm cuff due to size. Other places such as the forearm may need to be used. However, direct measurement of blood pressure via an indwelling catheter is recommended as there could be considerable hemodynamic changes during both induction and positioning the patient in the lateral thoracotomy position. Central venous access can be technically difficult in morbidly obese patients and the use of an ultrasound-guided method is recommended.

Positioning

A morbidly obese patient should never be allowed to lie supine when awake. When awake obese patients are placed in the supine position; there is increased mass loading of the ventilatory system, particularly on the thoracic and abdominal component of the chest wall. This produces a reduction in functional residual volume resulting in hypoxemia. The venous return also decreases due to compression of the inferior vena cava. Pelosi *et al.* found a linear relationship between the increase in BMI and the reduction in FRC.

Always preoxygenate the patient in the reverse Trendelenburg position. This will prolong the duration of safe apnea time after muscle relaxation for tracheal intubation. Another favorable position is the semi-Fowler position with the patient's upper body elevated 25–30°. In both positions the panniculus drops down and unloads the diaphragm, increasing the functional residual volume.

Changing to the lateral position requires additional physical help and equipment. Beanbags to support the patient in the lateral decubitus position may not sufficiently wrap around the patient due to their excessive girth and patients may need to be restrained with belts or tape across the pelvis. Supporting the head in the lateral, flexed position can be difficult due to a proportionally short neck. Care must be taken to avoid metal contact with any overhanging skin. All limbs should be fully supported and protected. Measurement of cardiac output is useful in patients with impaired ventricular function during one-lung ventilation.

Placement of double lumen tubes (DLT) and one-lung ventilation (OLV) in morbidly obese patients

Placement of double lumen tubes in morbidly obese patients could become difficult due to difficult laryngoscopy. A "difficult airway" has been defined as the clinical situation in which a conventionally trained anesthetist experiences problems with mask ventilation, with tracheal intubation, or with both. The incidence of difficult laryngoscopy and tracheal intubation may be as frequent as 7.5% in the normal surgical population. Difficult intubation due to inadequate exposure of the glottis by laryngoscopy is known to increase with increasing BMI, large neck circumference and Mallampatti scores of 3 or more. At present, there are no studies comparing the success of DLT placement in morbidly obese patients with normal-weight patients. In cases of difficulty, single lumen tubes with bronchial blockers could be used.

Use a large DLT to minimize airway resistance in morbidly obese patients undergoing OLV. Direct airway measurement is an accurate way of selecting a DLT rather than tube selection based solely on patient gender, height and weight.

Successful one-lung ventilation in morbidly obese patients in the lateral position is possible if the abdominal panniculus falls away from the body and unloads the dependent diaphragm.

Basilar atelectasis worsens following induction of general anesthesia. Positive end expiratory pressure can overcome this to some extent. In morbidly obese patients, ventilation with large tidal volumes does not improve oxygenation and can result in excessively high peak pressures during OLV. High peak inspiratory pressures due to restriction of the chest wall, reduced diaphragmatic excursion and the narrow bronchial lumen of a DLT can further limit volume-controlled mechanical ventilation during OLV. Pressure-controlled ventilation is a better mode as this maintains a sustained pressure during the breath to open up the alveoli.

Anesthetic agents

Morbidly obese patients have a higher proportion of adipose tissue and lower proportions of tissue water and lean body mass. These can cause differing patterns of drug distributions. The volume of distribution and clearance of propofol is increased in morbidly obese patients. The dose of propofol for induction and continuous infusion should be based upon actual body weight rather than calculated body weight. There is some evidence that prolonged use may be associated with slower recovery, but it is unclear whether extreme obesity contributes to the observed effect.

Atracurium and vecuronium both have a limited volume of distribution, but whereas vecuronium dosing is based on ideal body weight, the hyposensitivity to atracurium observed in obese individuals necessitates calculation of the dose on the basis of total body weight.

Studies by Juvin *et al.* and other investigators have demonstrated that post-operative recovery in morbidly obese patients is faster after shorter-acting inhalation anesthesia than propofol anesthesia especially after prolonged procedures. Rapid recovery is desirable to ensure early efficient coughing which can decrease the rate of post-operative respiratory complications.

The lipophilic benzodiazepines have a markedly increased volume of distribution and elimination half-life in morbidly obese patients. They should be used cautiously and avoided in patients with symptoms of obstructive sleep apnea.

Post-operative period

Early tracheal extubation after completion of a pulmonary resection lowers the risk of bronchial stump disruption and pulmonary air leaks secondary to positive-pressure ventilation. Tracheal extubation in a morbidly obese patient should be performed with the patient fully awake and sitting up to optimize ventilation. The patient should have a regular breathing pattern and good cough reflexes. Good pain relief is paramount in achieving this.

Epidural analgesia has proven advantages and can be delivered in either the lumbar or thoracic area, depending on operator comfort and anatomic ease. An experienced anesthetist is important in successful epidural placement in the morbidly obese patient. The anatomical landmarks may become difficult to identify due to excessive adipose tissue, but the midline can be easily identified by sitting these patients up. Paravertebral blockade can be as effective as epidural blockade and can be performed during the procedure under direct visualization of the thoracic cavity by the surgeon. Large doses of epidural opioids are best avoided in patients with proven or suspected OSA to avoid delayed respiratory depression.

Morbidly obese patients have a longer recovery time and a greater incidence of post-operative complications than normal-weight patients. These patients have a higher risk of post-operative atelectasis than normal-weight patients, which can persist beyond 24 hours after the end of the surgical procedure. The risks of venous and pulmonary thromboembolism are also greater in morbidly obese patients but outcome studies on obese thoracic surgical patients have not been performed. All obese patients must have mechanical and pharmacologic thromboprophylaxis. The "correct" dose of low molecular-weight heparins has not been established in obese patients.

FURTHER READING

- AAGBI. *Peri-operative Management of the Morbidly Obese Patient.* 2007. www.aagbi.org/publications/guidelines.
- Brodsky JB, Lemmens HJ. Tracheal width and left double-lumen tube size: a formula to estimate left-bronchial width. *J Clin Anesth* 2005; **17**: 267–70.
- Brodsky JB, Lemmens HJ, Brock-Utne JG, *et al.* Morbid obesity and tracheal intubation. *Anesth Analg* 2002; **94**: 732–6.
- Eichenberger A, Proietti S, Wicky S, *et al.* Morbid obesity and postoperative pulmonary atelectasis: an underestimated problem. *Anesth Analg* 2002; **95**: 1788–92.
- Juvin P, Vadam C, Malek L, *et al.* Postoperative recovery after desflurane, propofol, or isoflurane anesthesia among morbidly obese patients: a prospective, randomized study. *Anesth Analg* 2000; **91(3)**: 714–19.
- Pelosi P, Croci M, Ravagnan I, *et al.* The effects of body mass on lung volumes, respiratory mechanics, and gas exchange during general anesthesia. *Anesth Analg* 1998; **87**: 654–60.
- von Ungern-Sternberg BS, Regli A, Reber A, Schneider MC. Effect of obesity and thoracic epidural analgesia on perioperative spirometry. *Br J Anaesth* 2005; **94**: 121–7.

Chapter 22

Management of thoracic surgical emergencies

SAMEENA T. AHMED

The avoidance of thoracic surgical emergencies remains the goal of all thoracic surgery. Intraoperative prevention, prompt diagnosis and rapid correction is essential as thoracic emergencies can rapidly become fatal.

Tension pneumothorax

A pneumothorax refers to accumulation of gas in the pleural space resulting in collapse of the lung on the affected side. A tension pneumothorax is a life-threatening condition that occurs when the air within the pleural space is put under pressure; displacing mediastinal structures and compromising cardiopulmonary function. It can result from lung parenchyma or bronchial injury which acts as a one-way valve, allowing gas to move into the pleural space and preventing the free exit of that gas. Hypoxia results as the collapsed lung on the affected side and the compressed lung on the contralateral side compromise effective gas exchange. The venous return also falls as compression of the relatively thin walls of the atria impairs cardiac function. This results in hypotension and hemodynamic collapse.

Tension pneumothorax during one-lung ventilation

During one-lung ventilation, injury or compromise to the ventilated or dependent lung can progress rapidly to become a life-threatening emergency. Impaired dependent-lung ventilation usually presents as abnormal respiratory mechanics (i.e. increased airway pressure or decreased tidal volume), peripheral oxygen desaturation and cardiovascular instability with hypotension.

Thankfully, dependent-lung tension pneumothorax during thoracotomy and one-lung ventilation is not common. Literature review on this is limited to a few case studies.

Causes of tension pneumothorax during thoracic surgery

- Barotrauma from excessive tidal volume and high airway pressure may occur if the left-sided double lumen tube is positioned distally such that the entire tidal volume is directed to only one lobe.
- High tidal volumes and high airway pressures especially during re-expansion of the previously collapsed surgical lung.
- Air trapping within the dependent lung with hyperinflation and rupture of a subpleural bleb. On-line flow-volume monitoring might be useful in detecting the presence of air trapping. Smaller sized double-lumen can contribute to air trapping, especially during one-lung ventilation regardless of the patient's pre-existing pulmonary disease.

- Tracheo-bronchial disruption after placement of the double-lumen tube.
- Damage to the contralateral pleura during surgery.
- Lung injury after central venous catheter insertion or epidural placement.
- Pneumothorax may also occur after mediastinoscopy.

Management

The combination of abnormally high peak airway pressure, decreased tidal volume, decreased SpO_2 and hypotension during one-lung ventilation requires immediate intervention. Resumption of two-lung ventilation is required as the initial step. Airway obstruction from tube migration, secretions or blood should be ruled out with fiberoptic bronchoscopy. Typically, the fiberscope is passed through the tracheal lumen, first verifying a patent main stem bronchus, then confirming correct tube position by observing the bronchial cuff in the other main bronchus usually within 1 cm of the carina.

Fiberoptic bronchoscopy could show extrinsic compression of the main bronchus. When visualized through a bronchoscope, the airway will appear asymmetrically compressed for only a short segment with normal anatomy distal to the obstruction. With a tension pneumothorax, the major bronchi are circumferentially compressed, occluding the lobar orifices.

The surgeon should be alerted immediately to inspect for signs of dependent lung pneumothorax:

- Elevation of the dependent lung main stem bronchus.
- Mediastinal herniation into the operating hemithorax.
- An intra-operative cross-table lateral chest X-ray can further confirm the diagnosis.

The pneumothorax should be rapidly treated by chest drain insertion. The patient can be rotated to give the surgeon access to the dependent lung.

One-lung ventilation afterwards should be carefully monitored for tidal ventilation and airway pressures to prevent further lung injury.

Hemorrhage into the airways

The definition of massive hemoptysis varies widely in the literature, from 200 ml to 1000 ml/24 hours. Coughing up large amounts of blood is a terrifying experience for the patients. Conservative management of massive hemoptysis is associated with 75% mortality.

The main threat in the acute phase remains asphyxiation resulting from flooding of the airways and alveoli with blood. Maintenance of airway patency and control of bleeding are therefore the primary goals, followed by identifying the site and the underlying cause of bleeding. Correctly inserted double-lumen endotracheal tubes may achieve some of these goals through isolation of the affected lung and adequate ventilation of the non-affected lung.

Common causes of intra-operative airway bleeding are pulmonary artery catheter-induced perforation of a pulmonary artery, bleeding caused by vents inserted into the pulmonary artery or vein during pulmonary vascular repair and bronchial bleeding during lobectomy or pneumonectomy.

Bleeding into the tracheo-bronchial tree can come from either the bronchial or the pulmonary arterial systems.

Bleeding coming from the bronchial system results from neovascularization of the lung systemic vessels. This is induced by an inflammatory pulmonary disease or defect of the pulmonary arterial system. This can occur in bronchiectasis, suppurative lung disease, mycobacteriosis, etc. The blood vessels are endowed with a mural musculature wall, which is able to contract (arteriolar smooth muscle). Vasospasm of this network may be produced either by pharmacologic methods (vasoactive drug as vasopressin or aerosolized adrenalin) or by physical methods (bronchial ice-cold saline lavage) able to produce temporary slowing or cessation of the bleeding.

Bleeding from the pulmonary arterial system cannot be controlled by vasospasm as the wall of these vessels is thin with no active contraction. Bleeding is generally due to trauma or ulceration of the vascular wall caused by destructive processes such as necrotizing lung cancer or aspergillus cavitations. Bleeding can become fatal and surgical correction may be the only option.

Management

Initial resuscitation is aimed at stabilizing vital signs and oxygen saturation. All patients with massive hemoptysis should be monitored in the intensive care unit. Worsening hypoxemia is an indication of bleeding into the lungs and should be corrected with high-flow oxygen. The patient should be placed in a semi-Fowler's position. When the bleeding focus is already indicated by chest CT or angiography, they can be placed on lateral decubitus with the bleed side down to limit spoiling the non-bleeding lung. Systemic hypertension should be controlled if present.

Rigid bronchoscopy is recommended because of its greater suctioning ability and maintenance of airway patency. Fiberoptic bronchoscopy can be performed via a double lumen tube after the airway is secured. Profuse bleeding in the bronchi may render the localization of the hemorrhagic site very difficult when probing the affected lung with the fiberoptic bronchoscope. Instillation of vasoactive drugs (epinephrine diluted at 1:20 000) directly into the bleeding bronchus through the bronchoscope channel can decrease the hemorrhage. Endobronchial tamponade for bleeding control in massive hemoptysis was first introduced by Hiebert and colleagues in 1974. They occluded the bleeding bronchus with a balloon catheter via a rigid bronchoscope. Newer double-lumen balloon catheters are designed to pass through a fiberoptic bronchoscope. They have the advantage over the Fogarty catheter as administration of vasoactive drugs is possible through the second channel. Endobronchial tamponade should be used as a temporary measure in life-threatening situations. The catheter should be left in place while the patient undergoes other treatment modalities such as surgery, bronchial artery embolization, radiation or chemotherapy. Bronchial artery embolization is now considered the most effective non-surgical treatment in massive hemoptysis because of immediate and long-term results. Selective angiography should be performed to locate the bleeding bronchial artery before the injection of particles (polyvinyl alcohol foam, isobutyl-2-cyanoacrylate, absorbable gelatin pledget, or Gianturco steel coils). However, surgery remains the procedure of choice in the treatment of massive hemoptysis caused by specific conditions, such as hydatid cyst, thoracic vascular injury, bronchial adenoma and aspergilloma.

Myocardial ischemia and infarction with heart failure

In a series of 598 patients undergoing thoracic surgery for lung cancer, transient ischemic electrocardiographic changes were documented in 23 patients (3.8%). Myocardial infarction (MI) occurred in 7 (1.2%). Abnormal exercise testing and intra-operative hypotension were the strongest predictors for ischemic events. It is probable that a majority of patients undergoing thoracic surgical procedures will have some degree of CAD. The risk of peri-operative MI is estimated to be approximately 0.15% in patients without evidence of cardiac disease; however, in patients with a history of MI, the incidence of re-infarction during major noncardiac operations is estimated from 2.8–17.7%. Patients who have had drug-eluting stents for coronary revascularization should continue with their obligatory antiplatelet therapy requirements. This has implications for surgical bleed and placement of thoracic epidurals.

Herrington and Shumway reviewed the literature on MI in the post-thoracotomy period. Mortality rates ranged from 2.1–21%. However, the incidence of peri-operative MI was low (0.13%) in patients with no previous cardiac history to moderate (2.8–17%) in patients with a prior history of infarction. No association with present anesthetic techniques or duration of operative procedure with peri-operative ischemia or MI could be found, as long as patients were monitored invasively, baseline medication was continued, and peri-operative fluid administration was limited

Heart failure

Right ventricular dysfunction can occur due to alterations in the contractility and afterload. The right ventricular end-diastolic volume remains stable in the early post-operative period, however, significant increases may be observed on the first and second post-operative day.

Studies have found that pulmonary artery pressure and pulmonary vascular resistance only increase slightly suggesting that the rise in afterload is not the only factor. Despite changes in loading conditions, right ventricle (RV) end-diastolic volume and RV/work index remained within the limits of the preload recruitable/work relationship.

Both pulmonary embolism, occurring in 1%, and cardiac herniation are rare mechanisms that may cause RV dysfunction; especially the latter, which presents with a high mortality rate (40–50%). Although right heart failure is a substantial concern in thoracic surgery, there is no pre-operative predictive test for this complication at present.

Left heart failure is usually a consequence of impaired right heart function, either by decreasing left ventricular preload or by shifting the intra-ventricular septum resulting in a decreased left ventricular volume. Other causes of left ventricular dysfunction are acute myocardial infarction, pre-existing valvular disorders or cardiac herniation.

> **Box 22.1** Principles of managing heart failure
>
> Primary treatment of underlying cause.
> Hemodynamic support.
> Optimizing preload to the failing ventricles.
> Decreasing ventricular afterload by reducing systemic and pulmonary vascular resistance.
> Maximizing coronary perfusion through maintaining aortic pressures.
> Optimizing myocardial oxygen delivery.
> Limiting ventricular oxygen consumption.

During right ventricular ischemia and after infarction, the ventricle is unable to handle even "normal" loading conditions. Right ventricle ischemia leads to chamber dilation and an impaired diastolic function with a concomitant rise in RV end-diastolic pressure. The depressed right-sided output is followed by a decreased left ventricle (LV) preload. The elevation in RV diastolic pressure causes a shift of the interventricular septum toward an already under-filled LV. In the setting of limited pericardial compliance any right ventricular dilation leads to increased intra-pericardial pressures and an additional constraint on both the RV and LV filling. The consequence overall is a reduced cardiac output.

In contrast to the muscular LV, the thin-walled RV is poorly suited to compensate for acute increases in the afterload, such as in pulmonary embolism (PE). Here, the pulmonary arterial obstruction causes a sudden increase in the RV afterload. This increases wall tension and leads to chamber dilatation and impaired diastolic and systolic function. Acute tricuspid regurgitation resulting from RV dilatation and systolic dysfunction also leads to a diminished right-sided cardiac output and a reduction in the LV preload.

Clinical findings include systemic hypotension, tachycardia, tachypnea, cyanosis, elevated jugular venous pressure, a para-sternal heave and third-heart sound (Box 22.1). Hepatic enlargement and dependent edema are observed in acute-on-chronic heart failure. The current diagnostic options include ECG, chest radiography, cardiac biomarkers, echocardiography, cardiac MRI and right-heart catheterization.

Echocardiography provides a rapid and effective means for diagnosing heart failure as well as several associated conditions, including pulmonary hypertension, valvular disease, adult congenital heart lesions, cardiomyopathies and pericardial disease. Although transthoracic echocardiography provides direct visualization of the ventricles, technical and anatomic limitations may reduce its sensitivity and reproducibility, especially among the critically ill, mechanically ventilated patient population. In such patients, trans-esophageal echocardiography may provide a better assessment of cardiac structure and function.

Various modes of pharmacological inotropes and vasodilation have been described, including prostaglandins, beta-sympathomimetics, phosphorylase III inhibitors (milrinone), nitro compounds (nitroglycerin, sodium nitroprusside), alpha-adrenolitics (tolazoline, hydralazine), adenosine and inhaled nitric oxide. The vasodilators have all been used with variable degrees of success. Vasodilator treatment is often complicated by hypotension, which may compromise RV coronary blood flow and hence worsen RV failure.

With the exception of inhaled iloprost and inhaled nitric oxide, all other drugs currently used to treat pulmonary hypertension and increased PVR are non-selective vasodilators and may lead to systemic hypotension.

Dobutamine is primarily a beta-agonist with only minimal alpha-receptor agonist activity. This agent is, therefore, useful when further vasoconstriction is undesirable. At higher doses, dobutamine may induce tachycardia and atrial arrhythmias and increase oxygen demands.

Milrinone is a bipiridine phosphodiesterase III inhibitor. It has a positive inotropic action combined with a vascular smooth muscle-relaxing effect. The pharmacologic action of milrinone is mediated via the cAMP pathway; thus, it is independent of adrenoreceptor activity or increased catecholamine levels. Unlike dobutamine, milrinone does not increase oxygen demand. Beta-agonists can be combined with phosphodiesterase inhibitors to produce synergistic hemodynamic effects as well as increasing cAMP levels via two separate, and possibly synergistic, mechanisms.

Cardiac herniation

This is a catastrophic complication with a very high mortality. It is also a rare problem and hence can be overlooked easily. The most common cause is after intra-pericardial pneumonectomy with high negative pressures in the pleural cavity.

Symptoms usually develop within 24 hours, but late onset has been reported. In right-sided pneumonectomy the heart rotates counterclockwise around the axis of the vena cava, inducing a vena cava superior syndrome. In left-sided pneumonectomy the heart is strangulated by the pericardial sac, possibly causing superimposed myocardial ischemia. It can be precipitated by coughing, change of patient's position and application of negative pressure suction to the operated hemithorax.

Chest X-ray is useful in diagnosing right-sided cardiac herniation; it shows the heart in the right hemithorax. However the left-side herniation is more difficult to detect on an AP chest X-ray. A lateral rather than AP chest X-ray will show a posterior displacement of the heart.

Treatment

Immediate reduction of the herniation can be life saving. If the heart is not returned back into the pericardial space, the patient will not survive. As the patient is prepared for immediate re-exploration, negative pressure of the operated hemithorax must cease immediately. Positive pressure ventilation can further reduce preload and may not be safely tolerated. Spontaneous breathing should be maintained until the surgical team is ready. Mechanical ventilation with low peak airway pressures and PEEP should be used until the cardiac herniation is reduced.

Complications during mediastinoscopy
Major hemorrhage

Mediastinoscopy remains a widely used procedure for the staging of lung carcinoma and obtaining a diagnosis for diseases in the mediastinum. As mediastinoscopy involves dissection and biopsy of tissue in the superior mediastinum around the great vessels, there is always a risk of hemorrhage. All patients having mediastinoscopy should have large bore peripheral venous access. Direct arterial cannulation for measurement of blood pressure is also useful in these patients.

Major hemorrhage during mediastinoscopy is defined in the literature as bleeding greater than 500 ml; bleeding that requires a blood transfusion; and bleeding that requires exploration through a sternotomy or thoracotomy for control. There is no substitute for careful surgery. The operating surgeon must be familiar with the anatomic relationships within the mediastinum and perform careful dissection to expose the area of interest. When in doubt, needle aspiration should be performed to avoid direct biopsy of vessels. Despite these measures, major hemorrhage can occur. When a systemic artery is injured, digital compression or tamponade with the mediastinoscope is a first step in achieving control. If local measures fail to control bleeding or the patient develops persistent hemodynamic instability despite volume resuscitation, immediate surgical exploration through a median sternotomy should be performed. Sternotomy incision provides excellent access for injury involving the innominate artery or anterior surface of the superior vena cava. Injuries to the azygos vein or posterior aspect of the superior vena cava are more difficult to access through a sternotomy but can be managed with this approach. Cardiopulmonary bypass is often required and systemic anticoagula-

tion should be instituted as soon as the decision is made. Extensive posterior aortic injury may even require circulatory arrest to complete the repair.

If the mediastinum is distorted by prior surgery, radiotherapy or extensive, unresectable disease an extended period of packing can be used. The mediastinum pack may be left in place for 24 hours with the patient intubated and sedated. The following day, the patient returns to the operating room for removal of packing and re-exploration of the wound.

Superior vena cava obstruction

Obstruction of the superior vena cava was first described by Hunter in 1757. The common causes then were tuberculosis and syphilitic aneurysms of the ascending aorta. Nowadays, about 85% of all cases are attributable to cancer. The commonest cause is bronchogenic carcinoma (usually adenocarcinoma). Other malignant causes include fibrosis from central dialysis lines and pacing wires, lymphoma, mediastinal metastases (particularly breast and testicular cancer), Kaposi's sarcoma, and non-small-cell carcinoma. There is a higher risk of superior vena cava (SVC) obstruction when tumors are in the right upper lung because of the proximity to the superior vena cava.

The clinical presentation depends on whether the onset of obstruction is acute or chronic, and the amount of venous hypertension. Rapid obstruction does not allow for development of collateral vessels. This tends to be more rapid with tumors than infection. The patient might be unaware of this condition. Symptoms and signs include dyspnea, facial and neck swelling, and dry non-productive cough. Swelling of the face, neck, upper extremities and trunk should quickly arouse suspicion. The patient may have a feeling of fullness in the head that is worse when lying or bending forward. Edema may be present in the upper extremities. The skin of the upper chest, particularly on the right, will have collateral veins. Other signs include jugular venous distension, periorbital and conjunctival edema and suffused face.

Chest X-ray abnormalities include a widened mediastinum, upper lobe mass and pleural effusion. Computerized tomography (CT) with contrast can identify the site and amount of venous blockage. The SVC obstruction should be relieved prior to mediastinal surgery. Superior vena cava stenting provides the most rapid resolution of symptoms. Radiation therapy and chemotherapy can also relieve the symptoms. However this can take up to 3 weeks for symptomatic relief.

Anesthetic implications

Patients with SVC obstruction may have laryngeal edema and develop airway complications in the peri-operative period. This can become worse if the patient coughs on the endotracheal tube. Steroids and diuretics are often given to decrease edema and inflammation. Superior vena cava obstruction can compromise cerebral venous drainage. A head up position intra-operatively can be helpful in aiding cerebral venous drainage.

Intravenous anesthetic agents injected into the upper limb veins will have a slower circulation time. Central venous access, if required, should be via the femoral veins.

FURTHER READING

- Bardoczky G, d'Hollander A, Yernault JC, et al. On-line expiratory flow-volume curves during thoracic surgery: occurrence of auto-PEEP. Br J Anaesth 1994; 7: 25–8.
- Chan AS, Manninen PH. Bronchoscopic finding of a tension pneumothorax. Anesth Analg 1995; 80: 628–9.
- Decker J. Cardiac complications after noncardiac thoracic surgery: an evidence-based current review. Ann Thorac Surg 2003; 75: 1340–8.
- Endo S, Otani S, Saito N. Management of massive hemoptysis in a thoracic surgical unit. Eur J Cardio-Thorac Surg 2003; 23(4): 467–72.
- Flounders J. Superior vena cava syndrome. Oncol Nurs Forum 2003; 30(4): E84–8.
- Herrington CS, Shumway SJ. Myocardial ischaemia and infarction post-thoracotomy. Chest Surg Clin N Am 1998; 8: 495–502.
- Hiebert CA. Balloon catheter control of life-threatening hemoptysis. Chest 1974; 66: 308–9.
- Jougon J, Ballester M, Delcambre F. Massive hemoptysis: what place for medical and surgical treatment. Eur J Cardio-Thorac Surg 2002; 22(3): 345–51.
- Reed CE, Dorman BH, Spinale FG. Mechanisms of right ventricular dysfunction after pulmonary resection. Ann Thorac Surg 1996; 62: 225–32.
- Rowell N, Gleeson F. Steroids, radiotherapy, chemotherapy and stents for superior vena cava obstruction in carcinoma of the bronchus: a systematic review. Clin Oncol 2002; 14: 338–51.
- Urschel JD. Conservative management (packing) of hemorrhage complicating mediastinoscopy. Ann Thorac Cardiovasc Surg 2000; 6: 9–12.

Section 3 Post-operative management

Chapter 23

Peri-operative intravenous fluid management

SAMEENA T. AHMED

Management of intravenous fluids during thoracic surgery, particularly lung resection, is a longstanding contentious issue between anesthetists and thoracic surgeons. The anesthetists tend to focus upon the undesirable effects of tissue and organ hypoperfusion while the surgeons worry about problems caused by fluid overload and pulmonary edema after lung resection. The theory of fluid overload precipitating pulmonary edema was suggested by Zeldin *et al.* Their study consisted of ten patients who developed post-pneumonectomy pulmonary edema (PPO) and compared them with controls retrospectively. Increased amounts of intravenous fluids in the peri-operative period associated with large diuresis were found to be risk factors for this complication. However, fluid input and output data were only available for four of the ten cases. These authors further confirmed their findings in a dog model.

They recommended that "the most important thing we can do as surgeons in terms of recognising this problem is to watch our anaesthesiologists as they start loading the patients up with fluids."

Subsequent studies were unable to replicate this finding if the left heart filling pressures remained normal. Other investigators found no difference in the post-operative fluid balance of the patients who developed PPO and those who did not. These differences in the reported literature regarding fluid

administration and the potentially fatal complication of PPO may be due to variable clinical practices and poor quality of retrospectively collected data.

A cohort analysis of risk factors for acute lung injury (ALI) after surgery for lung cancer by Licker *et al.* demonstrated that excessive fluid infusion was a risk factor (odds ratio 2.9; 95% confidence interval). They found that patients who developed ALI had received in excess of 3 liters in the first 24 hours after surgery.

Effects of surgical trauma
Physiological changes resulting in fluid retention

Surgical trauma elicits a stress response via endocrine and inflammatory processes. The effects on fluid balance are mediated via the antidiuretic hormone (ADH), aldosterone and the renin-angiotensin II systems. It results in an increase in sodium and water retention with excessive potassium excretion.

- Increased ADH reduces diuresis and decreases plasma concentration of sodium.
- Increased aldosterone and renin-angiotensin activity leads to sodium retention and potassium excretion.

There is no evidence to suggest that renal function deteriorates in normovolemic patients with reduced urinary output. Protection of the fluid compartment is a physiological response to surgical stress.

Physiological changes to the lungs

Fluid homeostasis in the lungs is maintained via Starling's equilibrium via hydrostatic and colloid oncotic pressures.

- Net pressure pulling fluid out of the capillaries = hydrostatic pressure in the capillary minus the hydrostatic pressure in the interstitium.
- Net pressure pulling the fluid into the capillary = blood oncotic pressure minus the oncotic pressure of the interstitial fluid.

The net flow of lymph in the lungs is about 20 ml/min. This is reduced with pulmonary resection. As a result of fluid overload, the peri-bronchial and peri-vascular tissues become engorged. When the drainage capacity of the interstitial tissue is exceeded, the fluid passes into the alveoli, flooding them and causing pulmonary edema. The left and right lung lymphatic drainage in humans is different. On the right side, 94% of the lymphatic drainage is via the right hilum and 6% transverses the carina to drain into the left mediastinum. On the left side, 56% of lymph drains into the right superior mediastinum. Seventy-eight percent of the left lower lobe drains via the right side. Thus right pneumonectomy with associated trauma to the lymphatic drainage is more likely to cause post-pneumonectomy pulmonary edema than a left pneumonectomy.

Pulmonary capillary wall integrity is impaired after lung manipulation. This occurs after prolonged surgery, lung retraction, tissue handling and lung resection. The remaining lung tissue remains prone to acute lung injury which can progress to ARDS. A recent ARDS clinical trial network has concluded that conservative fluid management in the first 7 days after injury was better than liberal fluid administration. The patients had shorter duration of mechanical ventilation, better lung function and shorter duration of intensive care. This also points to the fact that maintaining normovolemia in the peri-operative period is preferred in thoracic patients. However, patients having large tissue dissection and mobilization such as esophagectomy and esophago-gastrectomy have higher fluid requirement than patients having pulmonary resection.

Early cardiac response to lung resection

The extent of acute cardiovascular changes after lung resection depends upon the amount of lung removed and underlying lung disease such as COPD. The resting mean pulmonary artery pressure and pulmonary vascular resistance tend to normalize after surgery. They increase by 30% with exercise in patients after pneumonectomy.

However, the right ventricular ejection fraction continues to fall in the first few days after surgery. This decrease in RV function is most likely due to an increase in RV afterload. This also occurs when supplemental oxygen is discontinued. Right ventricle dilation can also alter the left ventricular (LV) compliance by ventricular interdependence. Higher LV filling pressures may be required to maintain cardiac output.

The right ventricle fails if challenged by fluid overload, pulmonary edema, ALI or ARDS.

Assessment of the right ventricle pump functions in the thoracic surgical patient is often subjective and technically limited using transthoracic echocardiography. Thermodilution measurements of cardiac output using a pulmonary artery catheter have the advantage of supplying the pressures within the right heart. Unfortunately, the accuracy of these measurements is reduced in the presence of tricuspid valve regurgitation and exaggerated by acute increases in right ventricular afterload.

Fluid management in the peri-operative period

The aim of fluid management in thoracic surgical patients is to maintain normal hydration and accept reduction in urine output in the post-operative period.

Traditional anesthetic training dictates that replacement of fluid losses during surgery is the key target for peri-operative fluid management. Fluid losses are calculated based upon the length of fasting, surgical blood loss, evaporative losses from exposed body cavity and urine excretion. General anesthesia produces vasodilatation which further exposes these fluid deficiencies when the blood pressure drops. This is traditionally replaced by a large volume of crystalloid intravenous infusion. Thus intravenous fluid loading is considered indispensable.

However, fluid preloading and large intra-operative fluid administration are not evidence-based practice for best outcomes after surgery. Scientific evidence for an optimal fluid administration regimen resulting in adequate peri-operative organ function is lacking. Hence there is a large variation in the amount and type of fluid administered during surgery. Holte *et al.* demonstrated a reduction in pulmonary function within one hour of infusion of 22 ml/kg or 1–2 liters of normal saline. The same group further demonstrated that infusion of 40 ml/kg of Ringer's lactate over 3 hours reduced pulmonary function test up to 8 hours in healthy volunteers. This was also associated with weight gain. Infusion of fluid in excess of normal hydration can have physiologically adverse effects. These may be attributed to fluid accumulation in the interstitial tissues.

In the modern anesthetic practice, the recommended pre-operative fasting period is 4–6 hours. This does not normally cause intravascular hypovolemia.

- The measured evaporated fluid loss is 0.5 ml/kg. This increases to 1 ml/kg in patients having major surgery.
- Multiple clinical studies have demonstrated that fluid administration of more than 3 liters in the first 24 hours is a risk factor for ALI. Licker *et al.*

also demonstrated that patients who developed ALI received fluids in excess of 1 liter in the intra-operative period.

- Recommendations of standard anesthetic teachings for "third space fluid loss" of 6 ml/kg per hour in thoracic surgery are excessive. Except in unusual situations, it is best to assume there is no "third space" in the thorax.
- Unless there are other indications of developing renal failure, urine output greater than 0.5 ml/kg per hour is unnecessary in the normovolemic thoracic patient post-operatively.
- If increase in tissue perfusion is required in the peri-operative period, inotropes and vasoconstrictors should be used (guided by invasive monitoring) instead of risking volume overloading.

The management of acute right ventricular failure primarily involves inotropes, pulmonary vasodilators and inodilators. It is important to remember that vasoconstrictors such as pitressin and noradrenalin may be necessary to maintain right ventricular perfusion pressures.

Assessment of intravascular filling status in the peri-operative period

Blood pressure and cardiac filling pressures by themselves alone are a poor predictor of volume status. High central venous pressure can be due to right heart failure, raised pulmonary pressures, patient coughing on the endotracheal tube, etc. It does not reflect filling status. Similarly, raised blood pressure reflects raised systemic vasoconstriction and not adequate filling status. Findings from the physical examination such as mental status, blood pressure, heart rate, skin turgor, urinary output and serum electrolytes/osmolarity can be used in awake patients. However, these have their drawbacks in anesthetised patients.

Trends of mixed venous saturation from the SVC and PA can indicate a change in tissue oxygenation.

Peri-operative goal-directed intravenous fluid optimization using esophageal Doppler to guide an increase in cardiac stroke volume has demonstrated a reduction in hospital stay and fewer complications after colorectal surgery. There are no studies to indicate its effect on the thoracic surgical population.

However, less invasive measures such as systolic arterial pulse pressure variations in mechanically ventilated patients and central venous pressure variations in spontaneously breathing patients can distinguish between responders and non-responders to fluid challenges.

At present, there are no evidence-based data that using this can improve outcomes in thoracic surgical patients.

Blood transfusion in thoracic surgery

The purpose of blood transfusion in the peri-operative period (Box 23.1) is for the following:

- Improve oxygen carrying capacity.
- Improve hemostasis.
- Support circulating volume.

In addition to the well-known complications of blood transfusion, there is evidence that peri-operative blood transfusion can lead to immunosuppression. This effect can be detrimental in patients with cancer. Patients undergoing esophagectomy for cancer can have a worse outcome in terms of survival after receiving red cell transfusion.

Box 23.1 Factors that predispose to blood transfusion in thoracic surgery

Pre-existing anemia.
Previous thoracic operations.
Resection of inflammatory and infective disease processes.
Decortication of empyema.
Chest wall resection.

Patients with lung malignancies can become anemic pre-operatively. Anemia can be a sign of a more aggressive tumor. Studies have demonstrated that patients with non-small cell lung cancer (NSCLC) having a low hemoglobin concentration pre-operatively have a worse outcome. Early retrospective studies had concluded that patients with NSCLC having a blood transfusion did not have a good survival outcome. Berardi *et al.* studied the effects of peri-operative anemia and blood transfusion in patients undergoing lung resection for NSCLC. They demonstrated a worse prognosis in patients with hemoglobin less than 10 g/dl and those transfused in the peri-operative period. They concluded that anemia could be an important prognostic factor. Correction of anemia did not reduce the risk of relapse.

The immunosuppression induced by transfusion results from both an early unspecific pathway mediated by monocytes and a later phase induced one from increased suppressor T cell activity. Both effects are dependent on the number of transfusions. Blood transfusion has been shown to impair natural killer cell function and lower the CD4 to CD8 ratio. In addition, prostaglandin E_2 levels are increased after transfusion. This may result in a direct inhibition of interleukin-2 production from CD4 cells with subsequent effect, as interleukin-2 is obligatory for natural killer cell activity. Although it is not clear at a molecular level which factors influence immunosuppression after allogeneic blood transfusion in cancer surgery, there is good evidence that leukocytes in the blood mediate the effects seen.

Transfusion of fresh frozen plasma (FFP) has been linked with the development of pulmonary edema after lung resection. This might be due to the immunological effect. Fresh frozen plasma contains the complete (stable and unstable) humoral components of blood coagulation, fibrinolytic and complement systems. The presence of antibodies against the leukocytes in the FFP can trigger the onset of pulmonary edema. The activated leukocytes and granulocytes can migrate into the interstitial space between the alveolar and capillary endothelium resulting in capillary leaks and pulmonary edema. This is also known as transfusion related lung injury (TRALI). It is a variant of ARDS.

In the UK, all allogenic blood for transfusion is leukocyte depleted to minimize the possibility of new variant Creutzfeldt–Jakob disease transmission.

In the author's institute, there was not a strict blood transfusion policy for thoracic patients. However, care is taken to limit the amount of blood given peri-operatively. Other variables such as hemodynamic status and oxygen delivery are more important than an arbitrary hemoglobin concentration. Some patients will tolerate a lower hemoglobin level while others benefit from a transfusion.

Major blood loss may be unavoidable in operations. However, every effort should be made to reduce the amount of blood lost at the time of operation to an absolute minimum, and the importance of meticulous surgical technique cannot be overemphasized.

Other strategies that may limit the requirement of allogeneic transfusion include use of either pre-donated autologous blood or a Cell Saver. The use of a Cell Saver for transfusion of shed blood peri-operatively can increase the risk of dissemination of malignant cells and should be avoided in patients with cancer.

FURTHER READING

- Berardi R, Brunelli A, Tamburrano T. Perioperative anemia and blood transfusions as prognostic factors in patients undergoing resection for non-small cell lung cancers. *Lung Cancer* 2005; **49**(3): 371–6.

- Holte K, Jensen P, Kehlet, H. Physiologic effects of intravenous fluid administration in healthy volunteers. *Anesth Analg* 2003; **96**: 1504–9.

- Langley SM, Alexiou C, Bailey DH, Weeden DF. The influence of perioperative blood transfusion on survival after esophageal resection for carcinoma. *Ann Thorac Surg* 2002; **73**: 1704–9.

- Licker M, De Perrot M, Spiliopoulos A, *et al.* Risk factors for acute lung injury after thoracic surgery for lung cancer. *Anesth Analg* 2003; **97**: 1558–65.

- Pena CM, Rice TW, Ahmad M. Significance of perioperative blood transfusions in patients undergoing resection of stage I and II non-small-cell lung cancers. *Chest* 1992; **102**: 84–8.

- Slinger P. Post-pneumonectomy pulmonary edema. *Curr Opin Anesthesiol* 1999; **12**: 49–54.

- Van der Werff YD, van der Houwen HK, Heilmans PJM, *et al.* Postpneumonectomy pulmonary edema: a retrospective analysis of incidence and possible risk factors. *Chest* 1997; **111**: 1278–84.

- Waller DA, Keavey P, Woodfine L, Dark JH. Pulmonary endothelial permeability changes after major resection. *Ann Thorac Surg* 1996; **61**: 1435–40.

- Zeldin RA, Normadin D, Landtwing BS, *et al.* Postpneumonectomy pulmonary edema. *J Thorac Cardiovasc Surg* 1984; **87**: 359–65.

Chapter 24

General post-operative management

SAMEENA T. AHMED

Despite advances in the treatment of lung cancer, surgical resection remains the cornerstone of curative therapy. Post-operative management of thoracic patients continues to evolve. Recent scientific advances in surgical techniques, anesthetic management and peri-operative care have increased the number of operations performed in patients previously considered for palliative management only. Patients having thoracic surgery now have higher risks due to increased age, comorbidity, effects from smoking, debilitation and malnutrition due to cancer.

The immediate post-operative management of these patients has moved away from intensive care units to high dependency surgical step-down units with experienced nursing staff. Dedicated thoracic surgical high dependency units provide facilities for hemodynamic monitoring, oxygen therapy and ventilation support. The nursing and medical staff are trained to identify post-operative complication and manage chest drains.

General thoracic surgical wards should have a close working relationship with these purpose-designed high-dependency units. The emphasis on cost containment and effective use of resources in managing these complex patients remains a real challenge.

Thoracotomy even without surgical resection produces significant reduction in forced vital capacity (FVC) and functional residual capacity (FRC). Forced vital capacity and FRC can decrease to less than 60% of the pre-operative value on the first post-operative day. This eventually comes back to baseline after 2 weeks. Subsequent atelectasis predisposes the patient to shunting-related hypoxia and infection (Table 24.1). Respiratory complications (atelectasis, pneumonia and respiratory failure) can occur in 15–20% of the patients. Cardiac complications (arrhythmias and ischemia) occur in 10–15% of these patients.

Pre-operative management and changes in lifestyle can reduce post-operative morbidity and mortality. Smoking cessation can reduce post-operative morbidity. Patients should be encouraged to participate in smoking cessation programs often aided with nicotine supplementation and antidepressants. In 3–5 days, smoking cessation can improve ciliary clearance. Patients who have recently stopped smoking tend to have transient increases in sputum volume. Longer cessation can reduce secretions.

Pulmonary rehabilitation is also important. Pre-operative chest physiotherapy can reduce pulmonary post-operative complications in high-risk patients. Anesthetists rarely have the opportunity to assess these patients weeks before the surgery. In most cases, the anesthetist reviews these patients at the end of the referral chain. However,

Core Topics in Thoracic Anesthesia, ed. Cait P. Searl and Sameena T. Ahmed. Published by Cambridge University Press.
© Cambridge University Press 2009.

Table 24.1 Other post-operative complications.

Type of complication	Mechanism of injury	Presentation	Treatment
Vocal cord injury	Direct trauma or recurrent laryngeal nerve injury. (Especially the left nerve as it courses around the aortic arch). Surgeries that predispose to the injury include mediastinoscopy, anterior mediastinotomy, left pulmonary resection with subaortic dissection and resection of mediastinal tumors	Change of voice, aspiration of gastric contents and poor cough effort	Chest physiotherapy, withhold oral feed and change to nasogastric or parenteral feeding. In permanent damage, surgical repair of the vocal cord may be required
Atelectasis	Very common after thoracic procedures. This is due to poor pain control, inadequate cough and retained secretions. After left upper lobectomy the left lower lobe rises to fill the hemithorax and kinks the left bronchus as it passes under the aortic arch. After right upper lobectomy the horizontal fissure rises and rotates to a more perpendicular position resulting in twisting and kinking of the middle lobe bronchus. Lobar torsion can also present as atelectasis on the early chest X-ray	Patient presents with hypoxia, tachypnea, tachycardia, arrhythmias and signs of lung consolidation on auscultation of the chest. In lobar torsion, bronchoscopy will show an abrupt occlusion or twisted appearance of the airway	Measures to re-expand the collapsed lung with positive pressure breathing, chest physiotherapy. Bronchial toileting with rigid or fiberoptic bronchoscopy. Infections should be aggressively treated
Mediastinal and subcutaneous emphysema	This emphysema results from leakage of air under positive pressure (usually during coughing) into the subcutaneous tissue plane. The air then tracks along the mediastinal structures into the neck, head and chest wall. In some cases, it can track into the retroperitoneal space and the peritoneal cavity	It is identified clinically as crepitus in the neck, chest wall and head especially around the eyes	The problem is usually self-limiting unless there is pneumothorax, lung tear, bronchopleural fistula or esophageal injury/suture line leakage. Rarely, massive subcutaneous emphysema can cause airway obstruction requiring intubation. Positive pressure ventilation can worsen the subcutaneous emphysema
Pulmonary hypertension	Surgical resection of lung tissue decreases the cross-sectional area of pulmonary vascular bed. This normally compensated ability is reduced in patients with COPD	Right heart failure (high right atrial pressures with normal pulmonary capillary wedge pressures) and cardiac output state. Peripheral edema, hepatomegaly and oliguria	Aggressively treat reversible causes of pulmonary vasoconstriction (hypoxia, hypercapnea, acidosis, pain) Pulmonary vasodilators such as milrinone infusion. Optimize volume status with right heart catheter as well as echocardiographic assessment of left- and right-sided filling pressures

the anesthetist has a duty to identify the patients at higher risk and appropriately use peri-operative resources to improve outcome.

Early post-operative management

These patients should have routine post-operative monitoring (continuous ECG and oxygen saturation, intermittent non-invasive blood pressure or continuous blood pressure from indwelling arterial cannula) (Box 24.1). Oxygen supplement should be given to all patients in the recovery area and should be continued afterwards in the high dependency areas. The patient's trachea should be extubated after surgery as soon as they awake and can protect their airway. Secretion and blood retention in the airway are common after thoracic surgery especially after bronchoplastic procedures. Flexible fiberoptic bronchoscopy and bronchial toileting should be performed if there are excessive bloody secretions in the airway prior to extubation.

Laryngeal edema can occur after prolonged intubation with large DLTs, multiple attempts at intubation and rigid bronchoscopy. This presents as stridor after extubation. This is treated with sitting the patient in an upright position, intravenous corticosteroids and inhaled racemic adrenalin solution. If this is severe the patient may require re-intubation. If endotracheal intubation is necessary in the postoperative period, the double lumen tube (DLT) should be changed to a single lumen tube. Lung separation is not necessary in the post-operative period unless there is risk of lung soilage with blood or a need for differential lung ventilation. A DLT can cause airway trauma and edema. Airway toileting is difficult as the standard suction catheters are not long or narrow enough to pass through the lumen of the DLT.

Prevention of aspiration

Aspiration can be dramatic or an insidious event. It can happen in the early and late post-operative period. It is a life-threatening event in patients after pneumonectomy. Patients who have undergone high esophageal resection and anastomosis are prone to aspiration due to delayed recovery of airway reflexes. Oral intake resumes in most patients within the first 24 hours with the patient sitting upright. The swallowing mechanism and gag reflex must be assessed prior to oral intake.

Management of the chest drains

Chest drains allow the escape of air and blood from the thoracic cavity. Two drains are inserted after lung resection and a single drain after pneumonectomy. Classically, an apical drain removes air which rises to the apex and a basal drain removes fluids which gravitate downward. The chest drains are connected to an underwater seal drainage system. This is a simple and reliable one-way valve that allows air to escape from the pleura. Additionally, the volume fluid drained from the thoracic cavity can be collected and accurately measured. The underwater seal collection consists of a large diameter bottle with the chest drain terminating 2 cm below the water level. A short tube vents the bottle to the atmosphere. Low pressure suction is usually applied here (approximately -5 kPa). This system has been replaced by various disposable units that

Table 24.2 Causes of post-operative delirium after thoracic surgery.

Pre-operative	Intra-operative	Post-operative
Age	Prolonged surgical time	Sepsis
Male gender	Use of anesthetic agents with anticholinergic and antimuscarinic properties	Massive blood transfusions
Alcohol consumption	Hypotension	Inadequate pain control
	Embolism	Opiates
	Hypoxia	Sleep and sensory deprivation
	Massive blood loss	Abnormal serum electrolytes and glucose

incorporate the traditional functions into one plastic unit.

Chest drains should be monitored every 30 minutes for the first 2 hours and hourly during the first 24 hours. Documentation should include amount of fluid drained, color and presence of clots in the drainage. The water level in the water seal should be monitored routinely to check for evaporation. Fluctuations in the water level in the water-seal chamber of 5–10 cm, rising (during inhalation) and falling (during expiration), should be observed with spontaneous respirations. If the patient is on mechanical ventilation, the pattern of fluctuation will be reversed.

Chest drains must be removed by competently trained nursing staff. There is transient discomfort during the removal and the natural tendency is for the patients to draw in a sharp breath. Removal is undertaken during a Valsalva maneuver maintaining a positive intrapleural pressure. A purse string suture placed around the drain at surgery is tightened as the drain is removed.

Chest tubes after pneumonectomy

Surgeons usually place a single basal chest drain. This is connected to an underwater seal and left clamped. The clamp is released for 2–5 minutes every hour. This reveals excessive blood loss and centralizes the mediastinum. Suction should never be applied to the pneumonectomy drain. This can pull the mediastinum across and severely obstruct or totally occlude venous return to the heart with disastrous consequences. Pneumonectomy drains are usually removed the day after surgery if there is no active bleeding. This allows the pneumonectomy space to fill up with serosanguinous fluid at the rate of about two intercostal spaces per day. Over time, the remaining lung expands and pushes the mediastinum to the operated side, the diaphragm elevates and the intercostal spaces narrow.

Bleeding

Blood loss into the pleural space is expected but should not exceed 100–200 ml/hour. Thoracic high dependency units should have guidelines about management of bleeding and re-exploration of the chest. Facilities should be available for emergency surgery. Catastrophic bleeding occurs from pulmonary veins and arteries. Bleeding also occurs for vessels in the chest wall, mediastinum azygous vein and bronchial vessels.

Significant bleeding into the tracheobroncheal tree presents with hemoptysis. This is both frightening for the patient and the medical team. Treatment should comprise of maintaining the airway with clear and adequate ventilation. The DLT should be used to isolate the healthy lung while bleeding is controlled. Rigid bronchoscopy should be performed to tamponade the bleeding site with pledgets as soon as possible and clots removed. Emergency thoracotomy may be required.

Post-operative delirium after thoracic surgery

Post-operative delirium (POD) is defined as an acute change in cognitive status characterized by fluctuating levels of consciousness and inattention occurring after an operation (Table 24.2). It can occur up to 4 days after surgery. The incidence of post-operative delirium after thoracic surgery is reported to be 5–21%. It has been associated with major complications including increased morbidity, increased length of stay and poor functional and cognitive recovery.

Primary prevention is more effective than intervention and supportive measures. This includes correction of pain, hypoxia, sepsis, fluid balance and electrolyte deficiencies. Early ambulation should be encouraged. In 10–20% of patients with POD, no cause of delirium may be found. Pharmacological treatment may be essential to prevent injury to the patient and allow further evaluation. Haloperidol is a commonly used high potency antipsychotic agent in these patients. It is useful in treating delusions, paranoia and perceptual disturbances.

Chapter 25

Management of post-operative respiratory problems

CAIT P. SEARL

Although the exact incidence of post-thoracotomy respiratory failure is unknown, it can be estimated to lie between 5% and 15%. As many of these patients suffer from comorbid cardiopulmonary disease, pre-operative assessment is essential to try and help identify those patients at increased risk of developing post-operative respiratory failure. Efforts to minimize these risks include the aggressive use of analgesics. In the event of respiratory failure, the clinician must have a clear understanding of the underlying cardiopulmonary pathology, if any, and of the impact of the anesthetic and surgical procedures.

Extubation and airway concerns

The goal of extubation of the patient in the operating room remains the ideal. This avoids positive pressure ventilation or coughing against the endotracheal tube. Specific reasons to delay extubation include:

- Airway compromise due to bleeding or edema.
- Concurrent cardiac instability.
- An inability to protect against aspiration, e.g. due to severe neurological impairment.
- An open chest condition.
- Acute lung injury.

The silent aspiration of gastric contents following pulmonary resection remains an important complication. The continuation of endotracheal intubation in high-risk patients in this category for 24 hours post-operatively has been suggested to decrease both the risk of post-operative pneumonia and mortality. Lung separation techniques are generally unnecessary in the post-operative period and are usually replaced by a single lumen endotracheal tube if continued mechanical ventilation is required. Single lumen tubes are preferable as DLTs are more likely to cause airway trauma and edema due to their size; they are also more likely to displace and are difficult to suction through for bronchial toilet.

Post-operative respiratory failure

Life-threatening hypoxia or hypercapnia due to insufficient gas exchange and respiratory failure, after thoracic surgery is associated with a high incidence of mortality, accounting for around half of the mortality within the first 30 days of surgery. Table 25.1 lists potential causes of post-operative respiratory failure.

Ventilatory support after thoracic surgery

The twin goals of ventilatory support should be to provide inspiratory muscle assistance and rest while preventing the onset of muscle atrophy. To

Core Topics in Thoracic Anesthesia, ed. Cait P. Searl and Sameena T. Ahmed. Published by Cambridge University Press.
© Cambridge University Press 2009.

Table 25.1 Causes of respiratory failure.

Hypoxemic respiratory failure

Hypoventilation

Ventilation perfusion mismatch (normal pulmonary blood flow through poorly ventilated or edematous lung)

Focal consolidation	Collections (air, blood)
	Infection
	Inflammation
	Atelectasis
Edematous lung	Surgical injury
	Capillary leak
	Fluid overload

Right-to-left intrapulmonary/intracardiac shunts (e.g. due to a patent foramen ovale).

Abnormalities in alveolar oxygen diffusion.

Low fraction of inspired O_2.

Hypercapnic respiratory failure

Decreased function of muscles of respiration
Residual neuromuscular blockade
Surgical disruption
Structural/mechanical problems with the chest wall
Pneumothorax
Pulmonary contusion
Flail chest
Pain
Decreased central respiratory drive
Residual anesthesia or post-operative sedation
Central nervous system disease (e.g. peri-operative CVA)

that extent, the limitations of the various modes of mechanical ventilation must be appreciated as to their impact on patient ventilatory performance. Weaning from mechanical ventilation should be approached with an appreciation of the pathophysiological basis underlying the ventilatory failure, the factors responsible, and a rational approach to their improvement.

Following lung resection surgery, there is a concern that there will be an increased risk of bronchial anastomotic leaks or disruption with use of positive pressure ventilation. This risk needs to be balanced

against the need to optimize gas exchange to prevent hypoxemia and avoid hypercapnia. Intuitively the use of lower airway pressures is preferable, but there is no research evidence to identify a "safe" upper limit for positive pressure following lung resection. Avoidance of elevated airway pressures may be achieved by using reduced tidal volumes and pressure-limited modes of ventilation.

Non-invasive vs. invasive ventilation

Non-invasive positive pressure ventilation as management of acute hypoxemic respiratory insufficiency after lung resection has been shown to reduce the requirement for endotracheal intubation and "invasive" ventilation and to potentially reduce associated mortality. In situations where aspiration is not a concern and NIV is likely to be tolerated it may be preferable as to standard IPPV. Often NIV can be used as a step-up from cPAP. Our practice is to use cPAP to assist where atelectasis is thought likely to occur in combination with high-flow O_2/air, moving to NIV when hypercapnia is an additional problem.

Post-pneumonectomy pulmonary edema and acute lung injury

Acute lung injury (ALI)/ARDS is one of the main causes of mortality following surgery for lung resection. A survey of 1139 lung resections at the Brompton Hospital, London showed a frequency of 3.9% of ALI/ARDS, with these patients accounting for 72% of all mortality. The causes of ALI/ARDS following thoracic surgery remain unknown and are probably multifactorial. The clinical diagnosis of post-pneumonectomy pulmonary oedema so-termed by Zeldin in 1984 is unhelpful as the post-mortem changes in the lungs are indistinguishable from those of ARDS. The international consensus conference definitions should be used for ALI and

ARDS. Licker has further revised the diagnostic criteria as follows:

- Primary acute lung injury
  Within 0–3 days, no trigger.
  Associated with high intra-operative airway pressures, excessive fluid administration, pneumonectomy, pre-operative alcohol abuse.
- Secondary acute lung injury
  Develops between 3 and 12 days.
  Triggered by bronchopneumonia, aspiration, BPF, TRALI, etc.

The causative factors for ALI/ARDS post-lung resection include:

- Inflammatory injury.
- Ischemic-reperfusion injury.
- Oxidative stress.
- Surgical injury.
- Ventilation associated injury (particularly during one-lung ventilation).
- Oxygen toxicity.

A consideration of Starling's forces suggests the mechanism of edema formation: fluid movement across the wall of a capillary is dependent on the balance between the hydrostatic pressure gradient and the oncotic pressure gradient. This suggests the contributory factors to the development of ALI/ARDS following lung resection include damage to the lymphatic drainage; excessive fluid administration; and elevated pulmonary flow and pressures.

Prevention of ALI/ARDS post-lung resection
Fluid management

As discussed in Chapter 20, Zeldin implicated excessive fluid administration during the peri-operative period as the main cause of ALI/ARDS post-pnemonectomy (his post-pneumonectomy pulmonary edema). However, while excessive fluid administration is associated with poor outcomes,

it is unlikely to be the primary cause of ALI. The restriction of fluids in the management of established ALI as studied by the ARDS Net failed to show a survival benefit despite the patients having better oxygenation indices, reduced ventilator days and shorter ICU stays. A strategy for fluid administration during lung resection surgery might include a restrictive policy of replacing losses and avoiding hypovolemia, but using vasopressors to treat any hypotension secondary to anesthetic vasodilation rather than fluid administration. This recognizes that the maintenance of organ perfusion may help prevent causative inflammation as well as preventing end-organ damage. Administration of fluid may be guided by the measurement of central venous pressure and urinary output.

Ventilation strategies

Padley *et al.* reported that in ALI/ARDS following lobectomy, 8/9 patients had increased density in the non-operated lung. The peri-operative one-lung ventilation (OLV) may contribute to the development of ALI/ARDS through a combination of barotraumas, volutrauma and atelectrauma. Over-distension of the alveoli and damage to the alveolar eptthelium may occur due to air trapping, excessive tidal volumes and elevated inspiratory pressures. Mechanical difficulties with double lumen tubes have also been implicated as has the development of excessive intrinsic PEEP.

One-lung ventilation using similar lung ventilation strategies as adopted in the management of ALI/ARDS may be protective:

- FiO_2 to maintain $SaO_2 > 94\%$.
- PCV/CMV Plateau Pressure maximum of $25\,cmH_2O$.
- Respiratory rate 10–16 as guided by end-tidal CO_2, accepting $> 5\,kPa$ if necessary.
- Dependent PEEP as guided by the lower inflection point.
- cPAP to the operative lung if required.

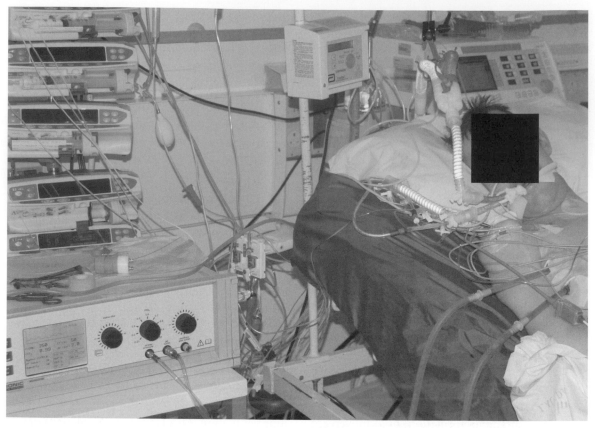

Figure 25.1 The use of a jet ventilator via the tracheal lumen of a DLT and conventional ventilation via the bronchial lumen in a patient with a BPF and empyema.

Further research is needed to evaluate strategies for risk reduction in patients undergoing lung resections who are at risk of acute lung injury.

Management of ALI/ARDS post-lung resection

As with ALI/ARDS in other situations, treatment is essentially supportive.

General supportive treatment

Nutrition: early enteral nutrition is desirable in all critically ill patients, but there is limited evidence to support an optimal composition.

Fluid management: fluid intake should generally be guided by central venous pressure and restricted where possible while maintaining adequate peripheral perfusion pressures.

Glycemic control: strict control of blood glucose gives a survival advantage to critically ill patients although there is no evidence to support this in ALI/ARDS patients.

Mechanical ventilation

Protective lung ventilation: The concept of *protective lung ventilation*, using tidal volumes limited to 6–8 ml/kg predicted body weight, has been widely adopted in recent years. The assumption is that this strategy avoids worsening volutrauma and atelectrauma and therefore triggers less inflammatory response. There is often a resulting decrease in clearance of CO_2. It appears in general that *permissive hypercapnia* is acceptable as a side-effect provided oxygenation is not compromised and the pH is maintained above 7.2.

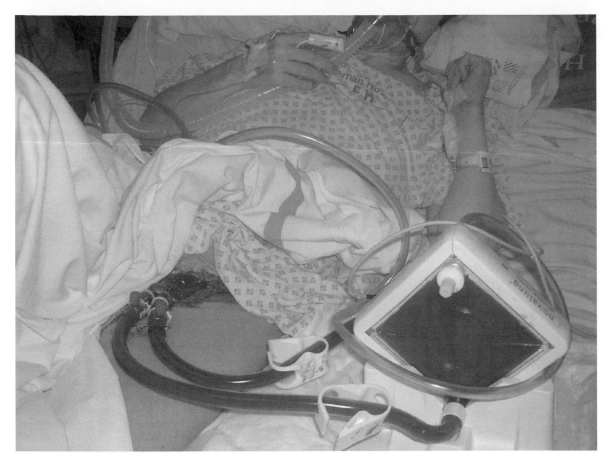

Figure 25.2 The Novalung device in situ treating hypercapnia in a patient with Type II respiratory failure.

Positive end-expiratory pressure (PEEP): Using PEEP improves oxygenation by increasing functional residual capacity by recruiting small airways and by decreasing the intrapulmonary shunting of blood through collapsed alveoli (decreasing ventilatory-perfusion mismatch). High levels of PEEP, however, can cause circulatory depression and lung injury from the over-distension of recruited lung units. At present it seems reasonable to set PEEP levels just above the lower inflection point of the static pressure-volume curve to optimize alveolar recruitment while minimizing shear stress.

High frequency techniques: These can be subdivided into high frequency positive pressure ventilation; high frequency jet ventilation (Figure 25.1); and high frequency oscillation. These use ventilatory rates between 60 and as high as 3000 cycles per minute. Using such techniques, areas with both low and high compliance (e.g. in a patient with both ARDS and a bronchopleural fistula) can be ventilated since gas distribution depends on airway resistance rather than compliance. Newer machines are able to provide humidification as well as ventilation. These techniques tend to be limited by hypercapnia.

Differential lung ventilation: Using a DLT it is possible to ventilate each lung separately using separate ventilators, ventilatory modes/settings, etc. The author has used conventional ventilators in this manner for example in patients with single lung transplants. The other setting for differential ventilation is where there is a need to stop spillage/contamination between lungs, for example in massive hemoptysis. I also have used differential ventilation allowing jet ventilation on the side of a BPF while conventionally ventilating the other lung.

Non-ventilatory adjuncts

Nitric oxide: Nitric oxide provides a short-lived beneficial effect on arterial oxygenation, intrapulmonary shunt and pulmonary vascular resistance. It has not been shown to provide any mortality benefit. The timing of NO administration has a critical impact on its therapeutic benefit for patients with acute respiratory illness. Administration before the onset of inflammation or very early in the inflammatory process may attenuate the inflammatory response in the lung and elsewhere in the body. Inhaled NO does not reduce the inflammatory response, once inflammation is already in process and may even increase peroxynitrite production causing increased oxidative damage.

Nebulized prostacyclin: Unfortunately nebulized prostacyclin has not been shown to provide survival benefit.

Pronation: Turning ventilated patients prone has been consistently shown to improve oxygenation in about 60% but to have no effect on overall outcome, that is mortality.

Extracorporeal CO_2 removal: Reducing the partial pressure of CO_2 and normalizing the pH can be achieved using extracorporeal percutaneously placed devices such as the Novalung (Figure 25.2). This lung-assist device is pumpless, relying on the patient's circulation to drive the blood from the femoral artery to veins via percutaneously placed cannulae through a heparin-bonded membrane, with removal of CO_2 using O_2 as the sweep gas.

ECMO: This is discussed in Chapter 22.

FURTHER READING

- Auriant I, Jallot A, Herve P, *et al*. Noninvasive ventilation reduces mortality in acute respiratory failure following lung resection. *Am J Respir Crit Care Med* 2001; **164**: 1231–5.
- DeHaven CB, Hurst JM, Branson RD. Evaluation of two different extubation criteria: attributes contributing to success. *Crit Care Med* 1986; **14**: 92.
- Kutlu CA, Williams EA, Evans TW, *et al*. Acute lung injury and acute respiratory distress syndrome after pulmonary resection. *Ann Thor Surg* 2000; **69**: 376–80.
- Licker M, de Perro M, Spiliopoulos A, *et al*. Risk factors for acute lung injury after thoracic surgery for lung cancer. *Anesth Analg* 2003; **97**: 1558–65.
- Padley SPG, Jordan SJ, Goldstraw P, *et al*. Asymmetric ARDS following pulmonary resection: CT findings – initial observations. *Radiology* 2002; **223**: 468–73.
- The National Heart, Lung and Blood Institute Acute Respiratory Distress Syndrome (ARDS) Clinical Trials Network: Comparison of two fluid management strategies in acute lung injury. *N Engl J Med* 2006; **355**: 317.
- Wang T, El Kebir D, Blaise G. Inhaled nitric oxide in 2003: a review of its mechanisms of action. *Can J Anesth* 2003; **50**: 839–46.
- Zeldin R, Normandin D, Landtwing D, Peters RM. Postpneumonectomy pulmonary oedema. *J Thorac Cardiovasc Surg* 1984; **87**: 359–65.
- 'Novalung – Solutions for Lung Failure' accessed at www.novalung.com.

Chapter 26

Extracorporeal membrane oxygenation (ECMO) and related technologies

JONATHAN HAYDEN SMITH

Extracorporeal membrane oxygenation (ECMO) is the use of an external oxygenator to replace lung function in cases of severe respiratory failure. The technique may be deployed for a period of several hours that may be extended to several weeks. The method was developed from the cardiopulmonary bypass circuit of the 1950s. The development of materials for oxygenators that were extremely durable meant that the bypass circuit could be adapted to support a patient when the lungs had failed. Silicone membranes which are non-porous with excellent gas exchange characteristics were best suited for use in the oxygenators for these extended periods of extracorporeal support.

The first survivor of ECMO was in 1971 in the USA. The technique was then developed and adapted by Dr. Bartlett and his coworkers. In the last 20 years the equipment and protocols are better understood so that the method can be applied by any appropriately trained group of physicians and nurses in an intensive care unit. The vast majority of the international ECMO experience is in children and much of that refers to the use of ECMO for the newborn infant.

ECMO is rarely used as a technique in thoracic surgery per se. It has been described as a useful technique in the treatment of tracheal injuries or stenosis and even as the pulmonary support of choice in lung transplantation. What follows is a description of how ECMO is currently applied to children and occasionally adults with pulmonary disease.

Rationale for the use of ECMO

The use of ECMO stems from the belief that ventilation of the lung with high pressures and high FiO_2 does cause trauma to the delicate tissues of the lung. It is not that all ventilation is harmful, but there are pressures and volumes that one can deliver to the lung that will compound the insult to the lung that occurs as a consequence of inflammation or infection. The same logic has led to the development of strategies of lower tidal volume ventilation and permissive hypercapnea. ECMO is a supportive therapy that provides oxygenation whilst the ventilator settings are reduced and should reduce ventilator induced lung injury. ECMO is only possible with systemic anticoagulation and the presence of an extracorporeal circuit. Whilst it has not been proven, most ECMO centers consider that there is a period of high-pressure ventilation beyond which the possibility of recovery of the lung with ECMO is small. In the UK neonatal trial the limit on duration of ventilation prior to the use of ECMO was 10 days; in the recent UK trial of ECMO for adult respiratory distress syndrome (Conventional ventilation or ECMO for Severe Adult Respiratory failure; CESAR), 7 days' ventilation was the cut-off after which a patient could not be admitted to the trial. If ECMO is to be part of the treatment algorithm for severe respiratory failure, the monitoring of the patient's response to treatment should be such that it is clear whether or not the patient fulfills ECMO criteria. This will allow appropriate referral of the patient once it is thought that the usual maneuvers in the intensive care unit have been completed within the eligible period.

Physiology

At the center of ECMO is the use of a membrane lung to allow oxygenation of the blood and CO_2 elimination. The physical principle used is that of diffusion. The oxygenator is designed so that the blood and gas phases are separated by a membrane and flow in different directions to give optimal conditions for gas exchange. The original membrane was silicone but in the last 5 years modified hollow-fiber oxygenators have been used in Europe; these have benefits in terms of a lower priming volume and a lower resistance to the flow of blood. The surface area of the oxygenator should be large enough so that given enough blood flow they can provide sufficient oxygen transfer to the blood to ameliorate the hypoxia that occurs as a consequence of profound pulmonary failure.

An understanding of oxygen delivery to the tissues is the key to an understanding of how ECMO works. Systemic oxygen delivery is the multiple of oxygen-carrying capacity and cardiac output (DO_2). This usually exceeds systemic oxygen consumption by a factor of 4 or 5 to 1. This excess is sustained by a combination of the cardiac output, the concentration of hemoglobin in the blood and the easy diffusion of oxygen and carbon dioxide across the alveolar capillary membrane in the lungs. A proxy measure for the adequacy of oxygen delivery in the face of continued oxygen consumption (VO_2) is the saturation of venous blood returning to the lungs. The saturation of blood in the pulmonary artery is the mixed venous saturation or $S\bar{V}O_2$. If the oxygen consumption increases sufficiently to erode

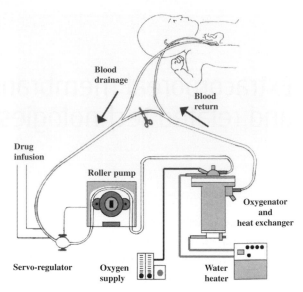

Figure 26.1 Schematic of the ECMO circuit for a newborn infant.

the reserve of the oxygen delivery then the pulmonary arterial and central venous saturations will fall. This proxy measure of the adequacy of oxygen delivery is nowadays commonly used in pediatric intensive care units and is always noted in ECMO circuitry. ECMO circuits are designed to augment the delivery of oxygen to the tissues by increasing the oxygen content of the arterial blood.

The technique of extracorporeal membrane oxygenation is designed to provide adequate oxygen delivery to the patient when the lungs have failed. To this end the system must:

- Have an adequate hemoglobin concentration (120–140 grams/l).
- Provide a blood saturation close to 100% at the output of the oxygenator.
- Be capable of delivering a flow such that the quantity of oxygen transferred to the patient in ml/min outstrips the needs of the critically ill subject in the intensive care unit.

The ECMO circuit (Figure 26.1), as with the cardiopulmonary bypass circuit, must be primed with an appropriate mixture of red cells, protein and crystalloid. The circuit can be connected to a

Table 26.1 A comparison of veno-arterial and veno-venous ECMO.

	VA ECMO	VV ECMO
Cannulation sites	RIJV, femoral veins, carotid, femoral artery or aorta	RIJV, femoral veins, either together or singly in terms of IJ double lumen cannulae
Usual PaO$_2$	60–150 mmHg	45–80 mmHg
Indicators of adequate oxygenation	SvO$_2$ measurement, lactate	Patient PaO$_2$, cerebral or tissue oximetry, lactate
Cardiac effects	Decrease preload and increase afterload	Negligible
Oxygen delivery capacity	High	Moderate
Circulatory support	Partial to complete	No direct effect, improved oxygenation often leads to improved cardiac function
Effect on pulmonary circulation	Reduced flow	Unchanged
Presence of right to left shunt	Reduced aortic saturations	Increased aortic saturations
Recirculation	None	Large impact on oxygen delivery

(Adapted from Fortenberry J, Pettignano R, Dykes F, *Principles and practice of venovenous ECMO in ECMO, Extracorporeal cardiopulmonary support in critical care*; ELSO 2005, used with permission).

patient in two modes, veno-arterial or veno-venous (Table 26.1).

Veno-arterial (VA) is the more traditional method; blood is drained from the great veins of the patient (usually SVC or IVC) and re-infused into an artery (in infants, most typically the carotid artery on the right side of the neck). The effect is to take venous blood of a low saturation and increase the saturation to 100% prior to infusing back into the arterial side of the circulation; this is a straightforward replacement of the patient's lack of pulmonary function. This gives pulmonary support but the interposition of a pump between the venous and arterial side of the circulation allows veno-arterial ECMO to be used for cardiovascular support as well; this is perhaps the most common reason for the deployment of ECMO currently.

The ECMO circuit can be connected in a veno-venous (VV) mode; in this configuration blood is drained from one part of the venous system, oxygenated and returned to another part of the venous system. The effect is to increase the venous satu-ration of caval blood prior to its passage through the pulmonary circulation. This can deliver enough oxygen to restore the oxygen transport in the patient to levels at which survival can be anticipated. It is a more elegant technique and avoids invading systemic arteries but results in a lower partial pressure of oxygen in the arterial blood. One must have a clear understanding of how much oxygen transport is increased by ECMO, particularly when using veno-venous ECMO.

Indications for ECMO

The usual indications for ECMO in the case of neonates are noted in Table 26.2.

ECMO is deployed on the understanding that the patient has a reversible condition. There must be an expectation that the lung injury the patient has sustained is self-limiting and reversible and that there has been no other injury to the patient that would preclude survival. Anticoagulation is required for ECMO and if there are contraindications to full anticoagulation ECMO should not be considered.

Table 26.2 The commonest diagnosis for the cohort of newborns that present for ECMO.

Indications for neonatal ECMO
Meconium aspiration syndrome
Neonatal respiratory distress syndrome
Group B streptococcal pneumonia
Persistent fetal circulation
Congenital diaphragmatic hernia

Life-threatening cardiac arrest or congenital anomalies have been considered contraindications.

In older children the usual indications for ECMO are viral and bacterial pneumonias complicated by ARDS. It is the author's view that patients with ARDS complicated by severe air leaks should be considered for ECMO in the absence of any contraindications.

Various ECMO criteria have been used. The most well known is the oxygenation index (OI).

The oxygenation index (Box 26.1) is a measure of the severity of ventilation (on the top line of the equation) and the effect of both ventilation and the right to left shunt on the PaO_2 in the child (on the bottom line). In the newborn infant the post-ductal PaO_2 is the result of two processes, the ability of the lungs to oxygenate the blood and the right to left shunt at ductal and atrial level that decreases the PaO_2 as a consequence of dilution with shunted pulmonary arterial blood entering the aorta

Box 26.1 The oxygenation index

MAP x 100 x FiO_2

Post-ductal PaO_2

MAP is the mean airway pressure in centimeters of water; FiO_2 is the fractional inspired oxygen concentration; the post-ductal PaO_2 (measured in mmHg) represents admixture of pulmonary arterial and aortic blood and reflects pulmonary dysfunction and degree of right to left shunting in the newborn.

(persistent fetal circulation). Despite its initial development in the care of newborns being considered for ECMO, the oxygenation index is used as a measure of the invasive nature of positive pressure ventilation for respiratory failure in adults. In newborns an OI of 40 or more over some hours is still considered a level that qualifies for ECMO. In older children and adults an oxygenation index of greater than 25 for some hours would suggest that ECMO might be considered.

The CESAR trial (**C**onventional ventilation or **E**CMO for **S**evere **A**dult **R**espiratory failure) of ECMO in adult respiratory failure has just finished recruiting at the time of writing. The criteria for ECMO in this trial was a composite of age between 18 and 65 years; severe but potentially reversible respiratory failure and a Murray score of greater than 3 or uncompensated hypercapnea with a pH of less than 7.2. The Murray score is a measure of lung injury based on the PaO_2/FiO_2 in mm of mercury on 100% oxygen; the number of quadrants of infiltration on the chest X-ray graded from 1 to 4; the level of PEEP on the ventilator and the measured compliance of the patient's lungs. Exclusion criteria were a period of high-pressure ventilation in excess of 7 days, intracranial bleeding or any other contraindication to limited heparinization.

Evidence for the efficacy of ECMO

ECMO has been extensively studied. The early negative studies had problems, as there was a lack of lung protective ventilation in the control limbs. Positive trials in newborns (Bartlett) and children (O'Rourke) used adaptive designs that were challenged at the time they were published. Both studies make interesting reading from the perspective of the early 21st century and helped promote the use of ECMO in the newborn population. It is worth noting that at the time of both those trials hyperventilation to hypocapnia was the conventional treatment for newborns with severe lung injury and persistent fetal circulation.

The UK collaborative ECMO study from 1993–1995 is one of the definitive randomized control studies in pediatric intensive care medicine. The conclusion that ECMO could produce one extra survivor for every three to four infants allocated to ECMO was highly significant and was not associated with an excess of morbid events. The ECMO cohort and their control group have continued to be studied and survivors in both limbs do have some long-term problems that may be referable to severe hypoxic illness in infancy. Subsequent work has confirmed that ECMO was cost-effective in this group of children.

The CESAR trial is the first randomized control trial of ECMO for adults in the current era. The trial design was such that ECMO in an ECMO center is tested against "best" conventional care in nine ECMO centers (these centers have to meet minimum criteria for provision of intensive care including lung protective ventilation and the ability to provide hemofiltration). This is a similar design to the neonatal trial. It is hoped that this will provide a level of evidence similar to the neonatal trial. There has been a debate on the applicability or not of ECMO to the adult patient with severe respiratory failure.

The Extracorporeal Life Support Organisation (ELSO) is the umbrella organization for centers that provide this therapy. It is based in the University of Michigan in Ann Arbor. It manages a database that is collated from member ECMO centers' submissions. The centers that are members of this organization contribute their own data so that the cumulative international ECMO experience can be surveyed, and summaries are produced twice yearly. As of July 2006 the total international experience contained in the ELSO database was just less than 25 000 patients with an overall survival of 65%; 60% of that total are neonates treated for respiratory failure; adults represent less than 4% of the total. Whilst this is a vast resource for the member centers it should be remembered that it is evidence and information available from ECMO centers alone rather than clinical trial data.

Equipment

The cannulae used for the provision of ECMO must be large enough to support the flow needed to allow adequate gas exchange. These modified bypass cannulae may be single lumen or double lumen depending on the form of ECMO deployed. In neonatal ECMO we would typically use a 12 or 15 French gauge double lumen cannula in the internal jugular vein to provide veno-venous support. An adult might have a 28 French gauge internal jugular venous cannula and a 24 French gauge femoral venous cannula for veno-venous support.

A typical newborn ECMO circuit is shown in Figure 26.1. The circuit packs are now produced commercially with the oxygenator and cannulae as separate components. Centrifugal or roller pumps may be used but the circuit design needs to be tailored to the pump employed. There must be a servo controller in the circuit such that when the venous drainage is curtailed (secondary to cannula obstruction or hypovolemia) the pump can be slowed or stopped. This prevents the phenomenon of *cavitation*, where gas can come out of solution if subjected to a negative pressure; air generated might then be pumped into the patient (air embolus). The servo controller is usually on the venous side of the circuit and is either a volume or pressure-sensing device. The venous side of the circuit contains many venous connections ("pigtails") used for infusions and blood sampling for the period that the child is on ECMO.

The oxygenators have been improved in recent years. In Europe the silicone oxygenators which made ECMO possible have been replaced with specially developed hollow-fiber oxygenators which require a lower priming volume and have a lower resistance than their predecessors (Figure 26.2). The new oxygenators also contain an integral heat exchanger.

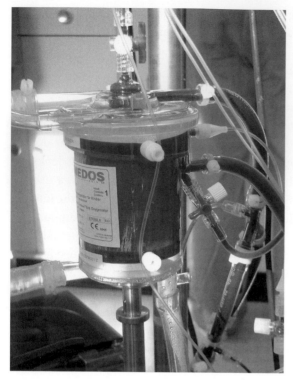

Figure 26.2 Modern Medos™ 2400 coated hollow fiber oxygenator, suitable for infants from 2–10 kg in weight.

Monitoring

Highly trained and experienced nurses are the mainstay of the care of the child on ECMO. The adjuncts that are used to monitor the child and the circuit are detailed below. These are in addition to the routine monitoring of a child on the PICU.

- An ultrasonic flow probe to check on flow to the patient; this validates the pump flow which most consoles calculate rather than measure.
- There are pressure monitors on both ends of the oxygenator that allow monitoring of the oxygenator's resistance to flow.
- A volume sensor ("bladder box") or pressure sensor to prevent cavitation and servo-regulate the pump.
- An in-line oximeter should always be attached to the venous limb of the ECMO circuit to monitor the saturation of the venous blood returning to the ECMO machine.
- Near infra-red spectrometers may allow assessment of local organ oxygenation at the bedside and are likely to be adopted widely in the ECMO community.

The routine method of assessing the degree of heparinization that is used for the child on ECMO is the activated clotting time (ACT). This automated near-patient investigation is produced by several different manufacturers whose ranges can vary. In the author's unit the Hemotec™ system is in use; the low range (LR) cartridges give a reading in normal circumstances of about 100 seconds. On ECMO we use an ACT of 180–220 seconds to represent adequate anticoagulation. The ACT is checked frequently immediately after heparinization and cannulation for ECMO and then 1–2 hourly thereafter during the course of the ECMO run.

The gas supply for the oxygenator usually comes from traditional flow meters and an oxygen blender.

The conduct of ECMO
Assessment

This often has to be made at a remote site from the ECMO provider but once a decision is made to offer ECMO on the previously cited criteria, the patient's transfer should then be arranged. Reversibility of the disease process and an absence of contraindications to heparinization are paramount considerations in this process. Once the adult or the child has arrived in the unit, reassessment of the patient's condition is usual prior to taking consent for and performing cannulation.

Cannulation

Once appropriate consent has been obtained cannulation is performed. The cannulation may be either percutaneous under ultrasound control or more commonly in the UK performed at open operation by surgical personnel. It is crucial that cannulae of an adequate size are selected such that the appropriate flow for the patient's weight and assumed cardiac output can be delivered. Anticoagulation is begun at the time of cannulation (100 U/kg of heparin) and the ACT checked; once the ACT is below 300 seconds an infusion of heparin (25 U/kg per hour) is begun and adjusted according to the ACT. It is not infrequent that cannulae might have to be repositioned or even added to and it should be made clear to the family of the patient that a combination of critical illness with some days of anticoagulation might lead to hemorrhage either at the cannula site or in the brain, gastrointestinal tract or even the lung.

Ongoing care

Whilst strategic decisions are made by the medical staff, the mainstay of ECMO is the care provided by the bedside nurses. With our current equipment two nurses are usually required to allow for care for both the patient and ECMO circuit. This 2:1 ratio can close beds elsewhere on the ICU but is necessary to provide safe care with adequate supervision of both the machine and patient. The general procedures of the intensive care unit are adhered to with regard to nutrition, fluid balance and infection control measures. Once the child is established on ECMO the ventilator can be turned down to what is termed "rest" settings; this is usually an FiO_2 of 0.21 and pressures of 20/10 cm of H_2O at a low rate. The skills required for looking after the circuit include understanding the basic science behind oxygen delivery; comfort with complex machinery; capability to perform CVVH; ability to remove patient from ECMO; and ability to operate the roller pump (or centrifugal pump) as per the local ECMO protocols. Successful units maintain a cadre of well-trained nurses who are able to do all these procedures and work to the protocols that guide the running of the ECMO circuit throughout the treat-

---

Box 26.2 General information on extracorporeal membrane oxygenation (ECMO)

ECMO is a modified form of cardiopulmonary bypass that can be used to support patients on the intensive care unit for many days.

Criteria for ECMO exist and can be calculated easily in most intensive care units; should a patient appear to qualify then the local ECMO center should be contacted to discuss suitability.

ECMO is a supportive therapy: the ability to rest the lungs and minimize the ventilator-induced lung injury allows pulmonary recovery.

ECMO has applications in neonatal and pediatric intensive care and may have a place in adult critical care medicine.

---

ment. Whilst some units, typically in the USA, have a small core of ECMO nurses it is our own practice to have everyone within the pediatric intensive care unit trained in the use of ECMO. Training in the unit must be regular with both induction and a regular review of skills. Without a structured training program "ad hoc" ECMO in the ICU will create risk and exhaust the perfusion resource in most hospitals. Recommendations on training and necessary drills to maintain experience are available from the extracorporeal life-support organization (www.elso.med.umich.edu).

The assessment of lung recovery during ECMO

ECMO is a supportive therapy (Box 26.2). The duration of bypass is determined by the rate of lung recovery from the initial injury; the age of the patient; the nature of the disease process; and probably the duration of high-pressure ventilation pre ECMO. Thus typically the newborn with pulmonary hypertension and severe meconium aspiration syndrome will be on ECMO for between 36–72 hours. An adult with ARDS secondary to pneumonia will be on ECMO for between 200–300 hours. With adequate in-unit experience and protocols, ECMO can be maintained for many days.

It is not unusual for the chest X-ray to "white out" immediately after ECMO has been initiated. This is most probably due to a combination of pulmonary inflammation, fluid infusion from the ECMO circuit and the cessation of high-pressure ventilation. Over the course of a successful ECMO run the lungs will clear radiographically and become more compliant. Weaning from ECMO has to be tested by reducing the oxygen supplied to the patient from the ECMO machine by reducing either the flow (in VA ECMO) or the gas flow across the membrane (in VV ECMO) so that the whole of the patient's gas exchange should be taking place in the lungs as the ventilation rate, FiO2 and ventilation pressures are increased. Once minimum flows have been achieved on the ECMO circuit and the blood gases are satisfactory the patient should be clamped off ECMO for several hours to trial the state of the patient's own lungs. If the patient is well, off ECMO and stable over some hours the cannulae should be removed.

Scenarios in which ECMO is useful
Neonatal respiratory failure with meconium aspiration

In meconium aspiration syndrome, the newborn has aspirated dense sticky meconium into the lungs during birth (Figure 26.3). This results in a complex of chemical pneumonitis, surfactant deficiency, respiratory obstruction and pulmonary hypertension. Should the neonate have an OI of 40 or more over some hours despite optimum therapy, ECMO should be considered. Once the infant has been cannulated for ECMO good tracheal toilet can be achieved with surfactant supplementation. The pulmonary hypertension resolves relatively quickly and the ELSO registry reports an aggregate survival for this condition of 94%. The registry reports an average run time of 129 hours. The UK experience

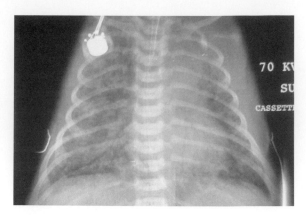

Figure 26.3 Chest radiograph typical of a newborn with meconium aspiration syndrome.

is that the usual run duration for meconium aspiration is 36–72 hours.

Adult respiratory distress syndrome (ARDS)

Adult respiratory distress syndrome is well recognized in the intensive care unit. Modern protocols for its management include careful fluid balance, conservative ventilation strategies with minimization of peak inspiratory pressures; tolerance of hypercapnea and attention to nutrition and cardiac output. Despite this some 30–40% of adults die with this syndrome. The CESAR trial is investigating the survival of adults with ARDS on ECMO. Their criteria include a Murray score of 3.5 or more and include many patients with a ratio of PaO_2/FiO_2 of less than 100. If the patient meets these criteria, has ARDS of a defined cause and the duration of prior ventilation is less than 7 days, ECMO should be considered. This is particularly so if the patient suffers from air leaks. The average run duration would be about 240 hours and one should expect a survival of between 50–60%.

Acute lung failure after pulmonary transplantation

Less than 5% of transplanted lungs fail to transfer sufficient oxygen immediately post-operatively and this can threaten the recipient's life. This is primary graft failure. It is not usually susceptible to ventilator therapy or inhaled nitric oxide. A number of lung transplant centers have demonstrated recovery from primary graft failure after a brief period of ECMO that is usually initiated during the first day after transplantation. This relatively rare phenomenon requires very clear unit protocols as regards the threshold for ECMO in this circumstance. The mode maybe either veno-arterial or veno-venous and it is usually performed via the femoral route. The duration of ECMO is between 3–7 days and a majority of the patients who survive will have lung function in their first year post-transplant that is comparable with those patients who were not treated with ECMO.

FURTHER READING

- Bartlett RH, Gazzaniga AB, Toomasam J, *et al.* Extracorporeal membrane oxygenation (ECMO) in neonatal respiratory failure: 100 cases. *Pediatrics* 1985; **76**: 479–87.
- *ECMO: Extracorporeal Cardiopulmonary Support in Critical Care*, 3rd edn. Van Meurs K, Lally KP, Peek G, Zwischenberger JB, eds. Available from ELSO.
- O'Rourke PP, Crone RK, Vacanti JP, *et al.* Extracorporeal membrane oxygenation and conventional medical therapy in neonates with persistent pulmonary hypertension of the newborn. *Pediatrics* 1989; **84**: 957–63.
- Oto T, Rosenfeldt F, Rowland M, *et al.* Extracorporeal membrane oxygenation after lung transplantation: evolving technique improves outcomes. *Ann Thorac Surg* 2004; **78**: 1230–5.
- The Acute Respiratory Distress Syndrome Network. Ventilation with lower tidal volumes as compared with traditional tidal volumes for acute lung injury and the acute respiratory distress syndrome. *N Engl J Med* 2000; **342**(**18**): 1301–8.
- UK Collaborative ECMO Trial Group. UK collaborative randomised trial of neonatal extracorporeal membrane oxygenation. *Lancet* 1996; **348**: 75–82.
- UK Collaborative Trial Group. Cost-effectiveness of neonatal extracorporeal membrane oxygenation based on 7-year results from the United Kingdom Collaborative ECMO Trial. *Pediatrics* 2006; **117**: 1640–9.
- www.Cesar-trial.org.
- www.elso.med.umich.edu/.

Chapter 27

Management of bronchopleural fistula

O. P. SANJAY AND SAMEENA T. AHMED

Bronchopleural fistula (BPF) implies that a communication exits between the pleural space and the bronchus. It can occur in 2% of patients after pneumonectomy. Several factors such as direct trauma, spontaneous alveolar rupture and necrotizing infection, poor wound healing due to nutritional status or adjuvant chemotherapy, iatrogenic causes such as puncture, laceration and barotrauma are cited as its etiology. The most significant risk factor for a BPF is mechanical ventilation after pneumonectomy where it is regarded as an ominous complication. The main factors that perpetuate BPF are high airway pressures which increase leak during inspiration, increased mean thoracic pressures throughout the respiratory cycle (PEEP, inspiratory pause, high I:E) which increase leak throughout the breath and high negative suction. All these factors tend to be present in patients with adult respiratory distress syndrome (ARDS) as they are necessary to support gas exchange and lung inflation.

Bronchopleural fistula occurs during mechanical ventilation in two general circumstances: as a localized lung or airway lesion (e.g. following trauma or surgery; complicating central line placement) or as a complication of diffuse lung disease (e.g. ARDS, *Pneumocystis carinii* pneumonia). Although most leaks are physiologically insignificant, BPF can predispose to atelectasis or inadequate inflation of ipsilateral or contralateral lung, interfere with gas exchange and predispose to pleural spread of infection. It can also prolong mechanical ventilation thus predisposing to additional morbidity.

Technical factors such as a long bronchial stump with excessive accumulation of secretions and subsequent infections can also predispose to development of BPF. The surgical technique of bronchial closure can also predispose to developing a BPF. There is no difference between hand-sewn or stapled bronchial closure and both techniques are performed at our institution. However, inadequate apposition of the bronchial wall, uneven sutures and loosely tied sutures can all lead to BPF. The bronchial stump should be covered with a flap made from the intercostal muscles, pleura or pericardium to reduce the possibility of BPF. Bronchial stumps on the left side tend to retract into the mediastinum and are less prone to developing BPF than the right side.

Clinical presentation

Bronchopleural fistula could clinically present as acute, subacute and delayed or chronic forms. In an acute presentation, BPF can be a life-threatening condition due to tension pneumothorax or asphyxiation from pulmonary flooding. The presentation

Core Topics in Thoracic Anesthesia, ed. Cait P. Searl and Sameena T. Ahmed. Published by Cambridge University Press.
© Cambridge University Press 2009.

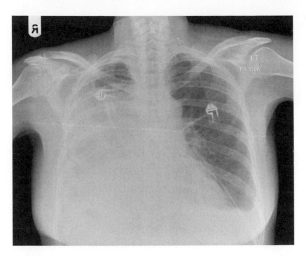

Figure 27.1 Chest X-ray of patient with BPF following right pneumonectomy.

is characterized by the sudden appearance of dyspnea, hypotension, subcutaneous emphysema, cough with expectoration of purulent material or fluid, shifting of the trachea and mediastinum, persistence of air leak, decrease or disappearance of pleural effusion on the chest X-rays. The subacute presentation is more insidious. It is characterized by wasting, malaise, fever, and minimally productive cough. The chronic form is usually associated with an infectious process. There is fibrosis of the pleural space and mediastinum preventing the mediastinal shift.

The consequences of BPF are

- Persistent pneumothorax.
- Inadequate ventilation.
- VQ mismatching.
- Infections of the pleural spaces.
- Inability to expand the remaining lung with PEEP.
- Inappropriate cycling of the ventilator.

Some BPFs are amenable to direct surgical repair (e.g. suture of bronchial tear; lobectomy for narcotizing pneumonia), but in most instances, resolution of the BPF depends on resolution of the primary disease process and of the pleural space infection (Figure 27.1).

Management

The first priority in managing a major pleural space infection is to protect the healthy lung parenchyma. If the patient is coughing copious sputum or blood, intubation is required to protect the remaining healthy lung. Keep the affected side in a dependent position as much as possible to prevent contamination of the other lung. Patients may be hemodynamically unstable with severe respiratory compromise and sepsis from the infected pleural space. These patients would require a high dependency level of care.

Bronchoscopy should be carried out as soon as possible to diagnose the fistula. Large fistulae can be easily detected. Small fistulae can be more difficult to find and the only indication could be movement/bubbling of secretions, necrotic tissue or granulation at the bronchial stump. Timing from surgery is critical when a BPF is diagnosed. The space should be urgently drained to reduce aspiration of fluid into the remaining lung. Appropriate antibiotics should be commenced to treat the empyema. Large chest drains are usually inserted to allow sufficient gas flows as air leaks could range from 1–16 liters/min. These should be placed in an underwater seal system without external wall suction.

Anesthetic considerations

The anesthetic goal is to control ventilation in the presence of an air leak:

- Achieve separation of the lungs.
- Prevent cross-contamination of the lungs.

If there is a chest tube in the affected side, it should be left unclamped prior to intubation. The chest should be drained before the induction of anesthesia to reduce the amount of purulent fluid in the chest cavity. If there is no chest drain present and the bronchi are not separated, there is a risk of tension pneumothorax developing when positive pressure ventilation is commenced. Hence intubation either

187

awake or after an inhalational induction with spontaneous ventilation should be considered. Anesthesia should be induced with the affected side in a dependent position, followed by prompt endobronchial intubation to isolate the healthy lung from contamination by purulent secretions from the affected side. Fiberoptic bronchoscopy is recommended to ensure accurate tube positioning. High frequency ventilation may be ineffective and even worsen the bronchopleural fistula if the healthy lung is not isolated.

Mechanical ventilation for patients with BPF

Mechanical ventilation may be required in patients. The air escaping through the BPF delays healing of the tract. It also accounts for a significant loss of tidal volume, jeopardizing the minute ventilation and oxygenation as this is an area of low resistance. The goal in promoting healing of the BPF has been the limitation of flow through the tract. Effective ventilation can be accomplished by using maneuvers that reduce the airway pressure, fistula flow and loss of tidal volume. These include:

- Limiting the amount of PEEP used during ventilation.
- Limiting the effective tidal volume.
- Shortening the inspiratory time.
- Reducing the respiratory rate.

In addition, the use of selective intubation of the unaffected lung with either the use of double lumen intubation and differential lung ventilation, or the use of independent lung ventilation and patient positioning are effective methods.

Ventilatory support should provide adequate inflation for the uninvolved areas of lung and assure adequate gas exchange. No single ventilatory mode or approach has been shown to be more effective than any other in treating patients with BPF. In the presence of a large air leak and difficulty in maintaining adequate ventilation, a ventilator

capable of delivering high inspiratory flow rates and large delivered tidal volumes may be required. Chest tube suction is necessary to evacuate continued gas leak, but the degree of suction exerts a variable effect on flow through the fistula.

The use of high-frequency ventilation (HFV) has been tried to overcome the limitations of conventional ventilation; however, reports have been conflicting. In general, HFV seems to be useful in patients with normal lung parenchyma and proximal BPF, while it is of limited value in patients with distal disease and parenchyma disease. High-frequency ventilation could be more applicable in conditions such as massive air leak due to BPF, which are difficult to manage by conventional ventilator modes.

Surgical closure of the BPF

This is only successful if the infection and inflammation around the stump resolves. It can take weeks or months to treat infections. Treatment options have expanded greatly in recent years. Empiric antibiotics are usually started before culture results have returned. The key to treating the infection is to eliminate the dead space. Chest tube drainage of the infected cavity and microbiological cultures are initial procedures. This may require multiple tubes or image-guided tube placement. Video-assisted thoracoscopy is useful for imaging to assess removal of fluid and necrotic tissues. Fibrinolytic therapy is often successful in fibrino-purulent or early organized cavities. A Clagett procedure, originally described by Clagett in 1972, is usually performed in patients with BPF as closed drainage is rarely sufficient. This involves resecting a large piece of rib, up to 6 cm in an anterior-lateral dependent position. This incision is more comfortable for the patient and allows easier subsequent change of dressings. A more permanent opening is obtained by performing an Eloesser flap whereby a flap of skin is rotated and stitched into the hemithorax after

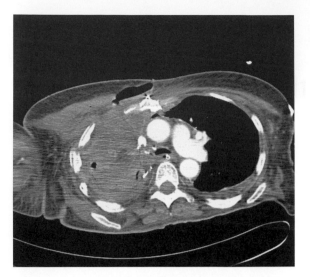

Figure 27.2 Computerized tomography scan showing that the myocutaneous flap extends into the right pneumonectomy space. The stump of the right main bronchus is in direct communication with the right pneumonectomy space collection.

Box 27.1 Guidelines for the management of bronchopleural fistula

To facilitate closure
  Use the lowest tidal volume that allows adequate ventilation.
  Use a ventilatory mode and settings that minimize peak and plateau pressures necessary to maintain adequate ventilation.
  Consider permissive hypercapnia to minimize inspiratory pressures and volumes.
  Minimize PEEP.
Consider independent lung ventilation (ILV) or high frequency jet ventilation (HFJV) in cases where a large air leak produces inability to inflate lung or failure to adequately oxygenate/ventilate.

rib resection. Some surgeons irrigate the pleural cavity continuously with saline or antibiotic solutions.

After sterilization of the cavity and stabilization of the patient, muscle flap reconstruction of the cavity may be performed (Figure 27.2). The nutritional status of the patient should be thoroughly assessed prior to any reconstruction.

The surgery aims to fill all residual space with muscle or omentum to decrease the risk of recurrent empyema. If the entire cavity cannot be filled, it may be partially obliterated by removing portions of overlying ribs. The patient should be followed closely as recurrence of the bronchopleural fistula or empyema cavity is possible.

In the future, tissue adhesives may play a more prominent role in the sealing of fistulae. Numerous case series involving fibrin sealants are reported in the literature. The most recent trend is to use bronchoscopic stents and sealants to limit contamination in combination with external drainage of the space.

REFERENCES

* Deschamps C, Pairolero PC, Allen MS, Trasteck VF. Management of post-pneumonectomy empyema and bronchopleural fistula. *Chest Surg Clin N Am* 1996; **6**: 519–27.
* Pierson DJ. Persistent bronchopleural air leak during mechanical ventilation. *Respir Care* 1982; **27**: 408.
* Powner DJ, Cline CD, Rodman GH Jr. Effect of chest tube suction on gas flow through a bronchopleural fistula. *Crit Care Med* 1985; **13**: 99–101.
* Sahn SA. Pleural disease in the critically ill patient. In Rippe JM, Irwin RS, Fink MP, Cerra FB, eds. *Intensive Care Medicine*, 3rd edn Boston, MA: Little Brown & Co., 1996; 720–36.

Chapter 28

Pain management after thoracotomy

ALEXANDER NG AND CHRISTINE TAN

The purpose of this chapter is to provide the reader with a concise account of locations of pain after thoracotomy, operative considerations relevant to pain relief and current methods of analgesia.

Neural input and locations of pain

Acute pain after thoracotomy occurs because of afferent nociceptive transmission along the intercostal, vagus and phrenic nerves. Patients experience incisional pain which is attributable to neural transmission along the intercostal nerves. In addition, there may be visceral pain which occurs as a result of vagal innervation of the thoracic organs.

Ipsilateral shoulder pain after thoracotomy is another frequent problem. It is of at least moderate intensity and occurs despite blockade of the suprascapular nerve supplying the shoulder. Deposition of local anesthetic in the interpleural space above the diaphragm does not obviate its occurrence. However, infiltration around the phrenic nerve with lidocaine has been shown to significantly reduce its occurrence.

Ipsilateral shoulder pain after thoracotomy is an example of referred pain rather than damage to the shoulder. Nociceptive transmission from the diaphragm and pericardium is transmitted along the phrenic nerve to the spinal cord. As the phrenic nerve and the shoulder have similar nerve roots, convergence of visceral and somatic impulses is possible. Ascending spinal pathways may be misinterpreted as emanating from the shoulder joint rather than from the diaphragm. This convergence-projection theory differs from the convergence-facilitation theory. In the latter, visceral diaphragmatic afferent input to the spinal cord would appear to cause the formation of an irritable focus rather than to be nociceptive per se. Shoulder pain arises because of amplification of previously innocuous somatic impulses from the shoulder.

Operative considerations

From the analgesic perspective, operative considerations may be classified into standard posterolateral thoracotomy and muscle-sparing thoracotomy.

Posterolateral thoracotomy

During a standard posterolateral thoracotomy, division of latissismus dorsi is required to obtain access to the intercostal space. In addition, it may be necessary to transect serratus anterior and trapezius.

Muscle-sparing thoracotomy

In a muscle-sparing thoracotomy, latissismus dorsi is not incised and serratus anterior is dissected and

Table 28.1 Analgesic techniques for thoracotomy.

Technique	Example
Thoracic paravertebral blockade	Bolus: bupivacaine 0.375% 20 ml Maintenance: bupivacaine 0.25% 0.1 ml/kg per hour
Intrathecal opioids	Single shot of: Morphine 500–750 µg With or without fentanyl 25 µg
Thoracic epidural analgesia	Bolus solution: bupivacaine 0.25% 10–20 ml Background solution: bupivacaine 0.1% with fentanyl 2–5 µg ml Background infusion rate 0.1 ml kg/hour Patient-controlled boluses possible e.g. 2 ml, with lockout interval of 30 minutes
Intravenous opioid by PCA	Morphine loading during surgery. 0.1–0.2 mg/kg Bolus: morphine 1 mg Lockout 5 minutes Maximum hourly dose 12 mg Background infusion, not required usually
Paracetamol	Regular paracetamol Dose 1 g, oral, rectal or intravenous
NSAIDs	Non-selective NSAIDs Oral or rectal diclofenac 150 mg per day in divided doses Selective NSAIDs (COX-2 inhibitors) Intravenous parecoxib 40 mg, twice daily
Others	Epidural clonidine Epidural epinephrine Oral gabapentin Intercostal nerve blockade Intravenous tramadol

Please note that the above drugs and doses are examples only. Drugs should be administered by appropriately trained and qualified practitioners. Adequate monitoring facilities are required.

reflected off the ribs to allow intercostal incision to be performed. However, the skin incision of a muscle-sparing thoracotomy traverses two to three dermatomes whereas that of the standard approach is over one dermatome. In addition, as access to the lungs is limited with a muscle-sparing thoracotomy, the ribs and surrounding tissue may have to be spread wider than when a posterolateral thoracotomy is performed. So, it can be seen that tissue trauma is not necessarily reduced after muscle-sparing thoracotomy.

Methods of analgesia

The main methods of analgesia are paravertebral analgesia, intrathecal opioids, epidural blockade and analgesic adjuncts (Table 28.1).

Paravertebral analgesia

ANATOMICAL CONSIDERATIONS

The paravertebral space is a potential wedge-shaped region, located lateral to the vertebral column and medial to the intercostal space. It lies posterior to the parietal pleura, and anterior to the superior costotransverse ligament and posterior intercostal membrane. Its superior and inferior borders are uncertain but it is probable that they extend from the occiput to the alar of the sacrum.

The paravertebral space contains spinal nerves that emanate from the intervertebral foramen. Components of these spinal nerves include their anterior and posteror rami as well as the white and grey rami communicantes. These spinal nerves are in continuity with the intercostal nerves, sympathetic chain, brachial plexus, lumbar plexus as well as the cervical and stellate ganglia.

Nociceptive conduction in the spinal nerves travelling through the paravertebral space is susceptible to blockade because of the lack of a surrounding fascial sheath. Owing to its close proximity, the ipsilateral sympathetic chain may be blocked by local anesthetics. In theory, bilateral neural blockade is possible because the paravertebral space is in continuity with the epidural space via the intervertebral foramen and also with the contralateral paravertebral space via the prevertebral and epidural spaces.

TECHNIQUE

To provide paravertebral analgesia for thoracic surgery, a Tuohy needle similar to that used for an epidural is used. Typically, this needle is inserted approximately 3 cm lateral to the spinous process of the fifth thoracic vertebrae, on the operative side. As the needle is advanced, it impinges on the transverse process of the six thoracic vertebrae. The needle is then redirected over the superior border of this transverse process to enter the paravertebral space which may be identified by loss of resistance to air or saline.

After bolus administration of local anesthetic into the paravertebral space, onset of blockade occurs after 40 minutes and ipsilateral analgesia

two dermatomes above as well as two dermatomes below the level of insertion is obtained generally. However, the degree of spread of local anesthetic is variable in the same patient and does not appear to be attributable to previous thoracotomy, age, sex, height and weight.

Variations on the above description of administration exist, for instance, placement of a catheter and multiple injections.

- Catheter: A catheter may be inserted percutaneously at induction of anesthesia or may be placed under direct vision by the surgeon during surgery. After surgery, a continuous infusion of local anesthetic may be administered.
- Multiple injections: Another variation of the single-shot technique at T5 or T6 is to administer local anesthetic in divided doses at T3 and at T7. The basis for this method is that thoracotomy at the fifth intercostal space involves dissection of muscle and skin innervated by dermatomes above and below T5 or T6. Blockade of afferent neural transmission in these dermatomes relies on adequate paravertebral cephalad and caudad diffusion of local anesthetic after a single injection. However, by administration of local anesthetic to the upper and lower dermatomal borders, it is thought that this uncertainty and hence possibility of insufficient analgesia may be obviated.

COMPLICATIONS OF PARAVERTEBRAL ANALGESIA

Complications of paravertebral analgesia are uncommon but they may include: pleural puncture, pneumothorax, vascular puncture, hypotension, dural puncture and Horner syndrome.

Horner syndrome is caused by blockade of the stellate ganglion or of the sympathetic preganglionic fibers of the first three thoracic vertebrae.

Clinical signs include ipsilateral ptosis, miosis, anhidrosis and enophthalmos. Rarely, it may coexist with harlequin syndrome contralateral to the side of paravertebral blockade. Harlequin syndrome comprises unilateral facial flushing as well as sweating, and thus it contrasts with the hemifacial pallor of Horner syndrome. Both syndromes are transient.

Intrathecal opioid analgesia

Intrathecal opioids provide effective analgesia after thoracotomy. Studies have been performed with preservative-free morphine, sufentanil and fentanyl. Morphine has a delayed onset but longer duration of action than fentanyl and sufentanil.

A combination of intrathecal morphine and sufentanil has been found to be associated with significant reduction in rescue morphine consumption as well as pain intensity at rest and coughing, for approximately 8–24 h, compared with placebo.

COMPLICATIONS OF INTRATHECAL OPIOIDS

After administration of intrathecal morphine 650 μg to 800 μg, the reported incidence of pruritus and nausea or vomiting is 37% and 25%, respectively. Other complications, for instance, respiratory depression, postdural puncture headache and epidural patch for dural puncture headache, occur in 3%, 0.54% and 0.37% of patients, respectively. Life-threatening respiratory failure, nerve injury and infection in the cerebrospinal fluid are most unlikely to occur.

Epidural analgesia

Epidural analgesia is often considered to be the gold standard for management of pain after thoracotomy. In this section, a number of issues will be discussed, i.e. epidural solutions; a comparison with other methods of analgesia e.g. intravenous morphine by PCA, paravertebral analgesia; and complications of epidurals.

EPIDURAL SOLUTIONS

The ideal epidural solution would be one which provides high-quality analgesia but without the adverse effects of its ingredients. Thoracic epidural solutions typically comprise local anesthetic, an opioid or a combination of both. Local anesthetics are associated with hypotension, motor blockade and urinary retention while opioids may cause pruritus, nausea and excessive sedation.

Administration of epidural bupivacaine and epidural morphine has been studied after thoracotomy. A bolus of 6–10 ml of bupivacaine 0.25% followed by an infusion of 3–5 ml of bupivacaine 0.25% for 3 days is as efficacious for analgesia as an initial dose of morphine of 2–3 mg and an infusion of morphine 0.1 mg/ml at 2 ml/h, for 3 days. However, the incidence of post-operative tachyarrhythmias may be significantly lower in patients who receive bupivacaine than in those who have morphine. This beneficial effect of epidural local anesthetic would appear to be attributable to sympathetic blockade and attenuation of a sympathotonic state during thoracic surgery.

The adverse effects of epidural local anesthetic and opioids are dose dependent and so the concentration of them would be one which provides effective analgesia with minimum adverse effects. The optimal concentration of bupivacaine in fentanyl 10 μg/ml has been studied. Bupivacaine 0.2% with fentanyl 10 μg/ml has been found to be associated with increased hypotension and use of vasopressors than bupivacaine 0.1% with fentanyl 10μg/ml. Pain relief is similar in both groups and so it may be seen that bupivacaine 0.1% is the more favorable concentration after thoracotomy.

In another clinical trial of patients after thoracotomy, epidural fentanyl at 2, 5 and 10 μg/ml in bupivacaine 0.1% have been compared. The solution containing fentanyl 5 µg/ml appears to be optimal because it provides better analgesia than that containing fentanyl 2 µg/ml and also because opioid-related adverse effects are reduced compared with fentanyl 10 µg/ml.

EPIDURAL ANALGESIA VS. INTRAVENOUS MORPHINE BY PCA

Epidural analgesia has been shown to provide better analgesia than intravenous morphine by PCA. In the recovery period, pre-incisional epidural bupivacaine 0.1% with morphine 0.05 mg/ml to 0.1 mg/ml is associated with significantly lower pain intensity scores at rest, cough and movement than intravenous morphine by PCA. In addition, the proportion of patients with pain lasting at least 2 months and of those with pain at 6 months would appear to be significantly lower in patients receiving epidural than in those who are prescribed intravenous morphine.

EPIDURAL VS. PARAVERTEBRAL ANALGESIA

It has been suggested that epidural analgesia may not be as effective as paravertebral blockade after thoracotomy. In a prospective randomized trial, patients who had epidural analgesia received 3 ml of bupivacaine 0.5% initially, 10–15 ml of bupivacaine 0.25% during surgery, 10 ml of bupivacaine 0.25% at the end of surgery and an infusion of bupivacaine 0.25% at 0.1 ml/kg per hour. The paravertebral group received bupivacaine 0.5% 20 ml prior to incision, bupivacaine 0.25% 20 ml at the end of surgery, and a continuous infusion of bupivacaine 0.5% at 0.1 ml/kg per hour. Pain scores at rest and on coughing, rescue morphine consumption, plasma cortical concentration and rise in glucose were significantly higher in patients receiving epidural analgesia than in those given paravertebral analgesia. Post-operative peak expiratory flow rates and oxygen saturation were significantly lower in the epidural group than in the paravertebral group.

These results have been supported, in part, by a systematic review and meta-analysis of ten randomized clinical trials comparing bolus and infusions of local anesthetics into the epidural and paravertebral spaces of patients having a thoracotomy. Pulmonary complications were significantly higher in patients receiving epidural analgesia than in those having paravertebral blockade. In addition, epidural analgesia was associated with significantly more urinary retention, nausea and vomiting, hypotension and block failure than paravertebral analgesia. However, both methods of analgesia appeared to be equally efficacious as there was no significant difference between them in post-operative pain scores and supplemental morphine consumption.

COMPLICATIONS OF EPIDURALS

As described above, epidurals are associated with adverse effects related to the components of the solutions administered e.g. pruritus, nausea and hypotension. In addition, infection is a complication and patients have an infrequent but serious risk of developing an epidural abscess. Neurological complications may occur after epidurals; they include dural perforation, radicular pain during epidural puncture or catheter insertion, transient post-operative radicular pain, peripheral nerve lesions, peroneal nerve palsy, other peripheral nerve lesions and paraplegia. To minimize this risk of neurological complications, there has been discussion that thoracic epidurals should be inserted awake rather than under general anesthesia.

Analgesic adjuncts

Simple analgesics such as NSAIDs and paracetamol have been shown to be useful for pain relief after surgery. In thoracic surgery, they have three main advantages:

- They have a systemic effect and thus can be used for the treatment of shoulder pain, especially in patients who have had an epidural.

- They minimize the dose of opioids used in epidurals, spinals and intravenous opioid infusions. Thus there may be a reduction in the possibility of respiratory depression in patients with partial lung function.
- They bridge the analgesic gap when either epidural or intravenous opioids are discontinued. The analgesic gap represents the period of time when patients may experience increased pain because a form of advanced analgesic support is discontinued and simple analgesics have not been commenced.

In addition, other analgesics, for instance, gabapentin may be useful for post-operative analgesia. Compared with placebo, oral gabapentin 1.2 mg, on the day of surgery and for a further 2 days has been associated with significantly lower pain intensity scores, paracetamol consumption, rescue epidural boluses, duration of epidural analgesia and motor block.

Key points

- Shoulder pain and chronic pain after thoracotomy are common.
- To manage pain after thoracotomy, the main methods of analgesia comprise epidural blockade, local anesthetics in the ipsilateral paravertebral space and intrathecal opioids.
- Analgesic adjuncts are useful e.g. paracetamol.

FURTHER READING

- Davies RG, Myles PS, Graham. A comparison of the analgesic efficacy and side effects of paravertebral vs epidural blockade after thoracotomy – a systematic review and meta-analysis of randomized trials. *Br J Anaesth* 2006; **96**: 418–26.
- Gwirtz KH, Young JV, Byers RS, *et al.* The safety and efficacy of intrathecal opioid analgesia for acute postoperative pain: seven years' experience of 5969 surgical patients at Indiana University Hospital. *Anesth Analg* 1999; **88**: 599–604.
- Mahon SV, Berry PD, Jackson M, Russell GN, Pennefather SH. Thoracic epidural infusions for post-thoracotomy pain: a comparison of fentanyl-bupivacaine mixtures vs. fentanyl alone. *Anaesthesia* 1999; **54**: 641–6.
- Oka T, Ozawa Y, Ohkubo Y. Thoracic epidural bupivavaine attenuates supraventricular tachyarrhythmias after pulmonary resection. *Anesth Analg* 2001; **93**: 253–9.
- Ng A, Swanevelder J. Pain relief after thorectomy: is epidural analgesia the optimal technique? *Br J Anaesth* 2007; **98**: 159–62.
- Richardson J, Sabanathan S, Jones J, *et al.* A prospective, randomized comparison of preoperative and continuous balanced epidural or paravertebral bupivacaine on post-thoracotomy pain, pulmonary function and stress responses. *Br J Anaesth* 1999; **83**: 387–92.
- Rowbotham DJ. Gabapentin: a new drug for postoperative pain. *Br J Anaesth* 2006; **96**: 152–5.
- Tan CNH, Guha A, Scawn NDA, Pennefather SH, Russell GN. Optimal concentration of epidural fentanyl in bupivacaine 0.1% after thoracotomy. *Br J Anaesth* 2004; **92**: 670–4.
- Tan N, Agnew NM, Scawn ND, *et al.* Suprascapular nerve block for ipsilateral shoulder pain after thoracotomy with thoracic epidural analgesia. A double blind comparison of 0.5% bupivavaine and 0.9% saline. *Anesth Analg* 2002; **94**: 199–202.

Chapter 29

Chronic pain after thoracic surgery

SAMEENA T. AHMED

Chronic pain after thoracotomy is defined by the International Association for the Study of Pain as "pain that recurs or persists along a thoracotomy incision at least two months following the surgical procedure." It is described as a burning, dysesthetic and aching sensation displaying many features of neuropathic pain. Chronic post-thoracotomy pain was first described by United States Army surgeons in 1944, who noted "chronic intercostal pain" in men who had had a thoracotomy for chest trauma during the Second World War. They identified the serious problem of chronic pain and the subsequent difficulty of rehabilitation and return to duty. This has not changed over time. Surgeons reported chronic thoracotomy pain in soldiers injured during Operation Freedom in Iraq. Intercostal nerve damage is responsible with no satisfactory treatment. Careful handling of the nerves can avoid unnecessary injury. There is no substitution for careful surgery.

Severe persistent pain affects 5% of patients post-thoracotomy. Dajczman *et al.* published the first data demonstrating the existence of chronic post-thoracotomy pain as a discrete entity. Studies have estimated the incidence of chronic post-thoracotomy pain at 11–80%. The wide variation in incidence can be attributed to differences in the definitions used to describe the neuropathic symptoms and the use of regular analgesia consumption. There is no objective evidence that the pain diminishes with time. Studies have looked at the occurrence of this pain beyond one year (50% of patients; Dajczman *et al.*), to beyond five after thoracotomy. The mean pain intensity (using a visual analog score) did not differ throughout this time. This pain can interfere with the patient's normal daily life. Even the gentlest stimulation can provoke intense and disabling pain. These patients require specialist intervention in chronic pain management clinics.

Clinical presentation

Neuropathic pain is different from acute pain due to tissue damage. The presentation, patho-physiology and management are more complex than with acute pain. The assessment of pain and other symptoms is required for diagnosis and subsequent management. The pain can occur spontaneously or as an abnormal response to stimuli. The pain can be continuous, intermittent or paroxysmal in nature. Patients have described it as "burning," "shooting" or "electric shock-like." Spontaneous paresthesia and dysesthesia can present as abnormal sensations such as "crawling," numbness and tingling. It is important to assess the duration and intensity of these sensations. Pain can also be evoked by

Box 29.1 LANSS scale for assessment of neuropathic pain

Symptoms associated with neuropathic pain
    "Pins and needles" (paresthesia) = 5 points.
    "Red skin" (autonomic changes) = 5 points.
    "Sensitive skin" (evoked dysesthesia) = 3 points.
    "Electric shock pain"; = 2 points.
    "Burning pain" (spontaneous dysesthesia) =
        1 point.
The physical assessment to identify allodynia
    Stroke cotton wool over the painful and the
        anatomically equivalent non-painful area.

    Numbness or tenderness in this area = 3 points.

    Altered pinprick threshold (PPT) by use of a 23
        gauge needle to assess perception of pinprick in
        the same areas.
A total score of 12 or more had a sensitivity of 79%
and a specificity of 100% for diagnosing
neuropathic pain

Box 29.2 Factors that can alter the occurrence of chronic post-thoracotomy pain

Strong association
    Benign esophageal disease.
    Post-operative radiotherapy.
    Cryoprobe neurolysis of intercostal nerves.
    Chest wall resections.
Weak association
    Malignant lung or esophageal disease.
    Rib resection
    Post-operative continuous extrapleural intercostal
        nerve block.

Box 29.3 Mechanism of intercostal nerve injury in thoracic surgery

Intercostal incision can damage the nerves directly.
Spreading the ribs with retractors can stretch the
    nerves.
Compression of the intercostal nerves with retractor
    and trocar.
Diathermy-induced injury.
Poorly repositioned rib fractures.
Costochondritis.
Intercostal neuroma, nerve entrapment and local
    infection.

non-painful stimuli such as gentle touch and pressure of clothing and temperature changes. Patients can become confused by the complexity of their pain symptoms and feel they might not be believed.

Specific pain assessment tools such as the Leeds Assessment of Neuropathic Symptoms and Signs (LANSS) scale (Box 29.1) may help in formalizing a diagnosis. This is a standardized bedside test that identifies patients in whom neuropathic pain mechanisms predominate.

Patients with complete disappearance of the superficial abdominal reflexes after thoracotomy experienced more severe acute and chronic post-operative pain than those in whom the reflexes are maintained and those whose abdominal reflexes do not recover 2–3 months after operation (i.e. who have an anatomical rather than functional deficit) are more likely to complain of pain. Patients with a higher degree of intercostal nerve impairment have greater post-thoracotomy pain (Boxes 29.2 and 29.3).

High consumption of analgesics during the first post-operative week is associated with a higher incidence of chronic post-thoracotomy pain. Adequate control of acute pain can reduce supra-sensitization by an effective afferent blockade of nociceptive stimuli.

Mechanism of neuropathic pain

The International Association for the Study of Pain defines neuropathic pain as "pain initiated or caused by a primary lesion or dysfunction of the nervous system." This may be in the peripheral or central nervous system, and frequently both systems are involved. The pain from thoracotomy originates via pain signals conducted by peripheral pain receptors, and the inflammatory process modulated by leukotrienes, nerve growth factor,

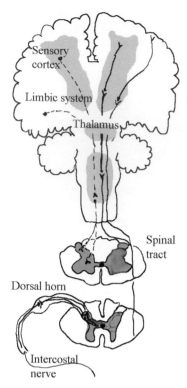

Figure 29.1 Pain pathways for thoracotomy pain. (*Courtesy of Mr. Richard Evans.*)

bradykinin, prostaglandins, histamine, and hydrogen ions. The afferent (incoming) pain signals reach the dorsal root ganglion, cross the synapse to a higher neuron horn of the spinal cord and connect in the dorsal horn with interneuron cells (Fig. 29.1). This is far from a simple, passive, one-to-one transmission. The afferent pain signal passes up the spinal cord via the spinothalamic tract to the thalamus. The pain signal is then sent to multiple locations in the brain. The interconnections within the brain are complex. They include both the sensory cortex and the limbic system, which gives the emotional aspect of chronic pain. The emotional aspect operates via the subcortical areas of the brain such as the thalamus, cingulate gyrus, hippocampus, amygdala, and locus ceruleus that interact to form the limbic system. The emotional component of pain is multifactorial. It is shaped by past experiences, genetic factors, general state of health,

psychologic distress, coping mechanisms, and beliefs and fears surrounding the pain. Of importance, thoughts and other sensations can influence the *sensory* pain input into consciousness as well as the *emotional* coloring of the pain sensation.

Chronic pain is not just a prolonged version of acute pain. The main neurotransmitter in the dorsal horn of the spinal cord is glutamate. This is a versatile molecule that can bind to several different classes of receptors especially the AMPA (alpha-amino-3-hydroxy-5-methyl-isoxazole-4-propionic-acid) receptors. In acute pain, the AMPA receptors activate the Na^+ and K^+ channels. In chronic pain, there is a persistent or large-scale release of glutamate. Repeated activation of AMPA receptors changes the membrane polarization. This removes the Mg^{2+} plugs in the Ca^{2+} channels. This marks the transition from acute to chronic pain. Activation of NMDA receptors has a number of important consequences:

- Activation of protein kinase C.
- Nitric oxide synthesis.
- Endorphin resistance.
- Release of substance P.
- Activation of NK1 receptors and triggering of c-fos gene expression which increases hypersensitivity.

The signal processing in the dorsal root ganglion and the dorsal horn is complex and only partly understood. They are influenced by the descending stimulatory and inhibitory signals from the brain and modulated by neurotransmitters. The process of increased excitability at the dorsal horn cell is termed as the "wind-up" phenomenon. The patient feels constant or increasing pain even when the peripheral stimulus has been withdrawn. These focal discharges stimulate adjacent uninjured nerve fibers, resulting in amplification of the pain impulses (peripheral sensitization). This leads to increased transmitter release causing increased response by spinal cord neurons (central sensitization).

Changes in acute pain

Changes in chronic pain

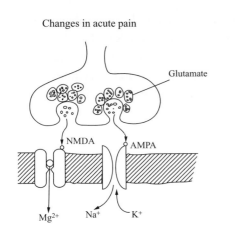
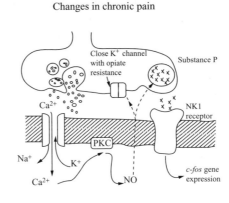

Figure 29.2 Changes in the nociceptor terminal in acute and chronic pain. (*Courtesy of Mr. Richard Evans.*)

Pre-emptive analgesia for prevention of chronic post-thoracotomy pain

Pre-emptive analgesia is a concept that originated from basic research indicating that an analgesic intervention is more effective if given before, rather than after, a noxious stimulus. The aim is to prevent central sensitization by blocking afferent C-fiber input from the periphery before the onset of a noxious stimulus.

Thoracotomy is known to produce high-intensity noxious stimuli sufficient to cause central sensitization. The area of post-thoracotomy pain is more discrete and largely restricted to the site of surgery. Hence, any benefit of pre-emptive epidural analgesia should, theoretically, be more apparent in thoracic surgery. However, the clinical usefulness of pre-emptive analgesia has remained controversial probably because of the wide variation in study conditions such as surgery, drugs and doses, routes of administration, treatment duration, and pain assessment methods used in different studies.

Katz *et al.* demonstrated that the intensity of early post-operative pain correlates with that of chronic post-thoracotomy pain. This led to the hypothesis that reducing acute post-thoracotomy pain with pre-emptive analgesia would result in a lower incidence of chronic post-thoracotomy pain. Obata *et al.* demonstrated that the use of thoracic epidural for post-operative pain control initiated before surgical incision reduced both the intensity of acute post-thoracotomy pain and the incidence of chronic post-thoracotomy pain. Other studies however, failed to show this benefit of pre-emptive epidural analgesia in preventing acute or chronic post-thoracotomy pain, both when taken individually or collectively in the form of a meta-analysis.

A larger randomized controlled trial, designed specifically to evaluate the effects of pain control prior to skin incision would be needed. It would need to be sufficiently powered to detect a significant difference in the severity of acute pain, as well as having an adequate follow-up period to detect any difference in the incidence of chronic post-thoracotomy pain (Fig. 29.2).

Surgical aspects of chronic post-thoracotomy pain

Thoracotomy involves incision of the skin and muscles to gain entry into the thoracic cavity. Serratus anterior and latissimus dorsi may be cut (muscle-cutting incision) or retracted (muscle-sparing incision).

Muscle-sparing thoracotomy has been devised to reduce soft tissue injury and acute post-operative pain and complications. However, this has not been uniformly validated in the literature. Some studies show there to be no difference in developing chronic pain. Others demonstrate that muscle-sparing thoracotomy was less painful at 1 week after thoracotomy.

The neuropathic nature of chronic pain led clinicians to devise techniques to preserve the intercostal nerves. The nerve above the incision is likely to get damaged during the rib retraction and the one below during chest closure. Rib resection could reduce intercostal nerve damage by avoiding trauma created by rib retraction or trocar insertion. However, periosteum scarring from rib resection might become a source of pain. All efforts should be made by the surgeon to avoid damaging the intercostal nerves, such as careful intercostal incision, minimal rib spreading and meticulous closure. At present, no surgical technique of thoracotomy can effectively prevent chronic post-thoracotomy pain. Hence, patients should be warned of the possibility of developing it.

Minimally invasive surgery should ideally reduce pain-related operative morbidity associated with classic open thoracic surgical techniques. Video-assisted thoracoscopic surgery (VATS) reduces both acute post-operative pain and analgesic requirements compared with both muscle-sparing and standard thoracotomy. However, comparative studies have not shown any difference in chronic pain occurrence between VATS and open thoracotomy. Intercostal nerve injuries and rib bruising or fractures can occur from trocar insertion or excessive torque of instruments during VATS. This may explain the similar incidences in the two groups.

Management of neuropathic pain

The management of post-thoracotomy chronic pain requires a multidisciplinary approach. The treatment plan should be individualized accordingly and include pharmacological (Table 29.1), interventional and behavioral options (Box 29.4). Adequate treatment requires a long-term commit-

ment from both patient and the medical team. The treatment goals should be realistic. Patients often hope for a "cure," but this is not always possible. Complete pain relief may not be achieved with treatment. A more realistic goal is to decrease pain to a tolerable level. This includes ability to self-care and to socialize. Specific goals should include activities the patient wishes to resume with pain relief. Effective treatment usually combines non-pharmacologic methods with medication.

Transcutaneous electrical nerve stimulation

Transcutaneous electrical nerve stimulation (TENS) is a safe and reversible therapy used widely by healthcare professionals involved in the management of pain. The theoretical rationale is to close the gate at the dorsal horn level. Electrodes may be placed over the corresponding peripheral nerve. The relief of pain is more effective when:

1. the pain is of peripheral origin;
2. the stimulated nerve lays superficially under the skin so it is accessible to electrical current delivered by external electrodes;
3. the electrodes are applied proximally to the causative lesion.

After thoracotomy procedures TENS can reduce opiate analgesic requirements and significantly lower pain scores.

Pharmacologic measures

Pharmacotherapy remains the mainstay for treating neuropathic pain. Different drugs used to treat neuropathic pain include topical agents, tricyclic antidepressants, anticonvulsants, opioids and non-opioid analgesics. The common underlying mechanism of action is to reduce neuronal hyperexcitability, either peripherally or centrally. Most drug trials have focused on the relief of pain, rather than the relief of symptoms such as allodynia, hyperalgesia, or the effect of treatment on the quality of

Table 29.1 Pharmacological interventions for post-thoracotomy chronic pain.

Agent	Mechanism of action	Side effects
Tricyclic antidepressants (amitriptyline)	Enhance the descending inhibitory pain pathway by inhibition of serotonin and noradrenaline uptake. They also improve the sleep pattern	Anticholinergic effects such as: dry mouth, constipation, urinary retention, sedation, weight gain, cardiac conduction
	The analgesic effect of TCA occurs at doses lower than the antidepressant effect	Abnormalities. Contraindicated in narrow-angle glaucoma
Anti-epileptic agents (gabapentin and pregabalin)	Limit neuronal excitation and enhance inhibition	Drowsiness, dizziness, fatigue, nausea, sedation, weight gain
	Act on voltage-gated ion channels (sodium and calcium channels), ligand-gated ion channels, glutamate and N-methyl-D-aspartate (excitatory) and GABA + glycine receptors (inhibitory). Pregabalin has a faster onset of action than gabapentin.	
Opioids	Strong opiates are not used as the first line agents in management of chronic pain. Morphine, fentanyl and tramadol are all used in different formulations. Tramadol works through a combined mechanism of weak mu receptor binding and the inhibition of serotonin and norepinephrine reuptake	Constipation, sedation, rebound pain (with short-acting opioids), and impaired cognition and drug tolerance
		Tramadol should be avoided in patients with a history of seizures or substance abuse
NMDA receptor antagonists (ketamine)	Epidural ketamine has been shown to reduce both acute and chronic post-thoracotomy pain by reducing central sensitization	Side-effect profile for epidural use not known as yet
	Ketamine also acts on opioid, cholinergic and MAO receptors	

life. This makes a comparative interpretation of the available treatments difficult.

Conclusion

Chronic post-thoracotomy pain is a serious and under-rated condition. Prospective observational trials are needed to determine the natural history of chronic post-thoracotomy pain and thus the extent of the problem. The neuropathic features strongly suggest that intercostal nerve damage is a major cause of post-thoracotomy chronic pain. Surgical techniques should be developed to preserve the intercostal nerves. This could reduce the incidence of chronic post-thoracotomy pain. Until this happens, patients need to be prepared for the real possibility of chronic post-thoracotomy pain.

Box 29.4 Non-pharmacologic management

Psychological techniques	Relaxation techniques may be helpful in some forms of neuropathic pain. Other techniques include meditation, cognitive behavior therapy, stress management and hypnosis.
Patient education	The evidence-base is lacking for this strategy. Logic would dictate however that an informed patient is more able to be involved in decisions about their care. This is certainly relevant in terms of compliance with treatment.
Acupuncture	Systematic evidence to support its use in neuropathic pain is lacking. There is some evidence that percutaneous nerve stimulation (PENS) which combines the techniques of acupuncture and TENS, may be helpful for some patients.

FURTHER READING

- Cohen SP, Griffith S, Larkin TM, *et al.* Presentation, diagnoses, mechanisms of injury, and treatment of soldiers injured in Operation Iraqi Freedom: an epidemiological study conducted at two military pain management centers. *Anesth Analg* 2005; **101**: 1098–103.

- Dajczman E, Gordan A, Kreisman H, *et al.* Long-term postthoracotomy pain. *Chest* 1991; **99**: 270–4.

- International Association for the Study of Pain: Subcommittee of Taxonomy. Classification of chronic pain. *Pain* 1986; **suppl. 3**: S138–9.

- Katz K, Kavanagh BP, Sandler AN. Acute pain after thoracic surgery predicts long-term post-thoracotomy pain. *Clin J Pain* 1996; **12**: 50–5.

- Maguire MF, Ravenscroft A, Beggs D, *et al.* A questionnaire study investigating the prevalence of the neuropathic component of chronic pain after thoracic surgery. *Eur J Cardio-thorac Surg* 2006; **29**: 800–5.

- Obata H, Saito S, Fujita N, *et al.* Epidural block with mepivacaine before surgery reduces long-term post-thoracotomy pain. *Can Anesth* 1999; **46**: 1127–32.

- Rogers ML, Duffy PJ. Surgical aspects of chronic post-thoracotomy pain. *Eur J Cardio-thorac Surg* 2000; **18**: 711–16.

Chapter 30

Arrhythmias after thoracic surgery

SAMEENA T. AHMED

Cardiac rhythm disturbances following thoracic surgery were reported by Currans in 1943. They continue to remain a common complication of thoracic surgery, especially pneumonectomy. The incidence varies between 11–28%. Arrhythmias appear within 3 days of surgery with a peak around the second day. The majority of them resolve spontaneously.

Supraventricular arrhythmias (atrial fibrillation, atrial flutter and supraventricular tachycardia) are commoner than ventricular arrhythmias. Atrial fibrillation accounts for 65–85% of all atrial arrhythmias after thoracic surgery. Arrhythmias after thoracic surgery serve as a marker for increased morbidity and mortality with increased length of hospital stay and use of resources.

Studies have reported an increase in mortality by 11–25%. This increases to 69% in patients who remain refractory to treatment. The increase in mortality has remained unchanged despite improvements in surgical techniques and post-operative high dependency care. However, the cardiac rhythm disturbances per se are not usually the direct cause of mortality in these patients. Early detection and aggressive treatment of hypotension to prevent further tissue/organ damage can improve outcome and prevent further arrhythmias.

Causes of arrhythmias after thoracic surgery

The sympathetic and parasympathetic nervous systems contribute to the cardiac plexus located close to the aortic arch and tracheal bifurcation. Surgical dissection especially during exposure of the hilum and mediastinal lymph nodes can damage the plexus. Vagal stimulation can also precipitate arrhythmias (Box 30.1).

Pulmonary resection produces an acute critical reduction of the pulmonary vascular bed. This can increase pulmonary vascular resistance and produce right heart failure with atrial distension and increased right ventricular volume. This can predispose to cardiac rhythm disturbances.

Pulmonary vein ligation is another risk factor. Electrophysiological studies have demonstrated that proximal parts of the pulmonary veins are covered by myocardial tissues. Surgical ligation of the pulmonary veins can produce a zone of ischemia and create a line of conduction blockage.

Major post-operative causes of arrhythmias are hypoxia, pain and electrolyte disturbances. Pain and hypoxia stimulate the sympathetic outflow and cause tachy-arrhythmias.

Studies have demonstrated that patients with high right ventricular pressure as determined by

Core Topics in Thoracic Anesthesia, ed. Cait P. Searl and Sameena T. Ahmed. Published by Cambridge University Press.
© Cambridge University Press 2009.

Box 30.1 Causes of arrhythmias after thoracic surgery

Hypoxia.
Vagal irritation.
Atrial distension.
Pre-existing cardiac disease.
Pulmonary hypertension.
Post-operative pulmonary edema.
Right heart failure.
Intra-pericardial resection.
Prolonged anesthesia and surgery.

cardiac echocardiography have a higher incidence of post-operative arrhythmias. This was not associated with an elevated right atrial pressure as measured with the central venous line. These findings were supported by another study that demonstrated diminished right ventricular function after pulmonary resection. There is an increase in the right ventricular end diastolic volume during the first two days after pulmonary resection. This corresponds to the period of high risk for development of arrhythmias. However, the pulmonary artery pressures and calculated pulmonary vascular resistance do not change. Whether this results from a myocardial alteration in right ventricular loading during the early post-operative period remains unclear.

Risk factors for arrhythmias

There are no specific risk factors for post-operative arrhythmias. Studies have attempted to assign a Cardiopulmonary Risk Index (CPRI) to patients pre-operatively to determine risks of cardiac complications. CPRI is a combination of the Goldman's Cardiac Risk Index and Pulmonary Risk Index which comprises obesity, cough, increased $PaCO_2$, reduced spirometric parameters, current cigarette smoking status and pre-existing reactive airways disease. There was no correlation found between CPRI and post-operative arrhythmias. However, pre-operative cardiac disease and $FEV_1 < 2.0$ cor-

related positively with post-operative arrhythmias. Other studies have demonstrated that age >70 years, extent of pulmonary resection and right-sided pneumonectomy are also independent predictors of post-operative arrhythmias.

Types of arrhythmias
Atrial fibrillation

Atrial fibrillation occurs from irregular beating of the atrium at 400–500 beats per minute. This results in multiple re-entrant circuits sweeping around the atrial myocardium. The sino-atrial node does not participate in the pace-making process. The atrioventricular node becomes incapable of transmitting these rapid impulses to the ventricles. The ventricles respond by beating irregularly. The ECG is characterized by a combination of absent P waves, fine baseline F wave oscillations, and irregular ventricular complexes. The ventricular rate depends on the degree of atrio-ventricular conduction, and it varies between 100 and 180 beats/min.

Fast atrial fibrillation may be difficult to distinguish from other tachycardia. The RR interval remains irregular, however, and the overall rate often fluctuates. Mapping R waves against a piece of paper or with callipers usually confirms the diagnosis.

Atrial flutter

This is not a common arrhythmia after thoracic surgery. It occurs via a re-entry circuit in the right atrium with secondary activation of the left atrium. The atrium contracts at a rate of 200–400 beats/min. This is seen on the electrocardiogram as flutter (F) waves. These are broad and appear as saw-toothed. They are best seen in the inferior leads and lead V1.

The ventricular rate depends on conduction through the atrio-ventricular node. Typically 2:1 block occurs. Identification of a regular tachycardia with this rate should prompt the diagnosis of atrial flutter. The non-conducting flutter waves are often merged with T waves and become apparent only if the block is increased. Maneuvers that induce transient atrio-ventricular block may allow identification of flutter waves. This arrhythmia is tolerated better than atrial fibrillation hemodynamically but ventricular rate control is required to allow better diastolic filling.

Multifocal atrial tachycardia

This tachycardia typically arises from an ectopic source in the atrial muscle. It produces an atrial rate of 150–250 beats/min (slower than that of atrial flutter).

Multifocal atrial tachycardia occurs when multiple sites in the atria discharge due to increased automaticity. It is characterized by P waves of different morphologies and PR intervals of different lengths on the electrocardiograph. The ventricular rate is irregular. It can be distinguished from atrial fibrillation by an isoelectric baseline between the P waves. It is typically seen in association with chronic pulmonary disease, commonly seen in patients undergoing thoracic surgery. Multifocal atrial tachycardia can degenerate into atrial fibrillation.

Treatment

The clinical importance of arrhythmia in an individual patient is related to the ventricular rate, the presence of any underlying heart disease, and the integrity of cardiovascular reflexes. Ventricular arrhythmia requires resuscitation of the patient from a hemodynamically unstable situation. The standard protocols recommended by the Resuscitation Council should be followed. These will not be discussed in detail here.

Atrial arrhythmia can be associated with identifiable factors such as hypoxia, electrolyte imbalance, administration of arrhythmogenic agents such as bronchodilators and catecholamines, myocardial ischemia and heart failure. Correction of these problems can alleviate the need for anti-arrhythmic medications in approximately one third of the patients (Box 30.2).

Box 30.2 Investigations for patients with arrhythmias

Serum electrolytes assay for potassium and magnesium.
Full blood count.
12-lead ECG.
Cardiac enzyme assay.
Arterial blood gases.
Microbiology sepsis screen.

Cardiovascular stability must be maintained to prevent tissue hypo-perfusion. If the patient has a low systolic blood pressure with a rapid ventricular rate, synchronized electrical cardioversion must be performed. Once the patient has cardiovascular stability, the next priorities can be to control the ventricular rate and reverse any correctable causes of atrial arrhythmias.

Drug treatment of supra-ventricular arrhythmias

The major issues in management of patients with AF are related to the arrhythmia itself and to prevention of thromboembolism. The two fundamental methods to manage the arrhythmia are to restore and maintain sinus rhythm, or to allow AF to continue and ensure that the ventricular rate is controlled.

The ventricular rate in patients with supraventricular tachy-arrhythmias can be controlled with drugs such as:

1. Beta-blockers (esmolol, metoprolol).
2. Calcium channel antagonists (diltiazem, verapamil).
3. Class III anti-arrhythmic agents (amiodarone, ibutilide) have been used with satisfactory results although there are different opinions.

Beta-blockers are preferred in patients with ischemic heart disease. They may be relatively contraindicated in patients with proven bronchospastic lung disease, congestive heart failure, severe sinus bradycardia or high degree AV-block.

Amiodarone has been used in recent studies in the management of patients with supraventricular arrhythmia with great success. Ciriaco *et al.* reported a 90.9% success in establishing sinus rhythm with no side-effects. The most common side-effect was bradycardia (< 50 beats per minute). This occurs in 13.5% of the patients.

In contrast Van Mieghem *et al.* reported that amiodarone may be implicated in the development of adult respiratory distress syndrome after lung surgery, especially pneumonectomy.

Anti-arrhythmic drug prophylaxis

There have been various attempts to prevent post-operative arrhythmias after thoracic surgery. Agents such as digoxin, amiodarone, diltiazem and beta-blockers have all appeared in the literature ranging from randomized prospective trials to case reviews. The results have not been positive universally. It is unclear whether prophylactic treatment against post-operative atrial arrhythmias improves clinical outcomes or shortens hospital stay using rate control or rhythm control agents.

Prophylactic digitalization has been attempted several times in the past using various combinations of pre- and post-operative digoxin administration. There was no difference in the occurrence of arrhythmias in the patients who were digitalized. The toxic effects of digitalis and the difficulty of assessing adequate digitalization in patients with normal heart function are the principal arguments against its prophylactic use in thoracic surgery.

Other studies have demonstrated the effectiveness of beta-blockers and class III anti-arrhythmic agents (amiodarone, ibutilide) in reducing the atrial fibrillation incidence after cardiac operations (valvular surgery, coronary artery bypass grafting). Amar *et al.* published a large, randomized control trial which demonstrated that diltiazem prevents atrial fibrillation after major thoracic operations.

Lanza *et al.* demonstrated that low-dose oral amiodarone prophylaxis significantly reduces the incidence of atrial fibrillation after pulmonary resection. More randomized control trials are required to test the prophylactic effects of these drugs to confirm these results in patients after major thoracic non-cardiac operations.

FURTHER READING

- Amar D, Roistacher N, Rusch VW. Effects of diltiazem on the incidence and clinical outcomes of atrial arrhythmias after thoracic surgery. *J Thorac Cardiovasc Surg* 2000; **120**: 790-3.
- Asamura H, Naruke T, Tsuchiya R. What are the risk factors for arrhythmias after thoracic operations? A retrospective multivariate analysis of 267 consecutive thoracic operations. *J Thorac Cardiovasc Surg* 1993; **106**: 1104-10.
- Atlee JL. Perioperative cardiac dysrhythmias: diagnosis and management. *Anesthesiology* 1997; **86**: 1397-424.
- Ciriaco P, Mazzone P, Canneto B. Supraventricular arrhythmia following lung resection for non-small cell lung cancer and its treatment with amiodarone. *Eur J Cardiothorac Surg* 2000; **18**: 12-16.
- Fuster V, Ryden LE, Asinger RW. Guidelines for the management of patients with atrial fibrillation. Executive summary. A report of the American College of Cardiology/American Heart Association. Task force on practice guidelines and the European Society of Cardiology Committee for practice guidelines and policy conferences (Committee to develop guidelines for the management of patients with atrial fibrillation). *Circulation* 2001; **104**: 2128-50.
- Haisaguerre M, Jais P, Shah DC, Takahashi. Spontaneous initiation of atrial fibrillation by ectopic beats originating in the pulmonary veins. *N Engl J Med* 1998; **339**: 659-66.

- Lanza LA, Visbal AL, De Valeria PA. Low dose oral amiodarone prophylaxis reduces atrial fibrillation after pulmonary resection. *Ann Thorac Surg* 2003; **75**: 223–30.
- Ommen SR, Odell JA, Stanton MS. Atrial arrhythmias after cardiothoracic surgery. *N Engl J Med* 1997; **336**: 1429–34.
- Van Mieghem W, Coolen L, Malysse I. Amiodarone and the development of ARDS after lung surgery. *Chest* 1994; **105(6)**: 1642–5.
- Von Knorring J, Lepantalo M, Lindgren L. Cardiac arrhythmias and myocardial ischemia after thoracotomy for lung cancer. *Ann Thorac Surg* 1989; **48**: 33–7.

Index